Recent Advances in Neurodegeneration
http://dx.doi.org/10.5772/intechopen.71995
Edited by Antonella Borreca

Contributors

Taosheng Huang, Zhuo Li, Jesse Slone, Lingqian Wu, Nibaldo Inestrosa, Juan Zolezzi, Sussy Bastias-Candia, Cristina Cereda, Matteo Bordoni, Valentina Fantini, Orietta Pansarasa, Sidharth Mehan, Jeremiah Ogbadu, Mamtaj Alam, Rishabh Jhanji, Devesh Agarwal, Shakshi Sharma, Aakriti Garg, Tarun Kapoor, Ramit Sharma, Raju Paudel, Urvashi Langeh, Pallavi Duggal, Kajal Rajdev, Khadga Raj, Shivani Verma, Himanshi Khera, Antonella Borreca

Notice

Statements and opinions expressed in the chapters are these of the individual contributors and not necessarily those of the editors or publisher. No responsibility is accepted for the accuracy of information contained in the published chapters. The publisher assumes no responsibility for any damage or injury to persons or property arising out of the use of any materials, instructions, methods or ideas contained in the book.

First published in London, United Kingdom, 2019 by IntechOpen
IntechOpen is the global imprint of INTECHOPEN LIMITED, registered in England and Wales, registration number: 11086078, The Shard, 25th floor, 32 London Bridge Street
London, SE19SG – United Kingdom
Printed in Croatia

British Library Cataloguing-in-Publication Data
A catalogue record for this book is available from the British Library

Additional hard and PDF copies can be obtained from orders@intechopen.com

Recent Advances in Neurodegeneration, Edited by Antonella Borreca
p. cm.
Print ISBN 978-1-83881-233-1
Online ISBN 978-1-83881-234-8
eBook (PDF) ISBN 978-1-83881-235-5

RECENT ADVANCES IN NEURODEGENERATION

Edited by **Antonella Borreca**

We are IntechOpen,
the world's leading publisher of
Open Access books
Built by scientists, for scientists

4,300+
Open access books available

117,000+
International authors and editors

130M+
Downloads

151
Countries delivered to

Our authors are among the

Top 1%
most cited scientists

12.2%
Contributors from top 500 universities

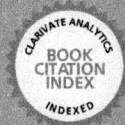

Interested in publishing with us?
Contact book.department@intechopen.com

Numbers displayed above are based on latest data collected.
For more information visit www.intechopen.com

Meet the editor

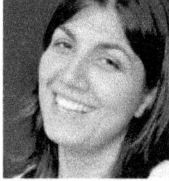

Antonella Borreca is a molecular biologist specialized in the field of neuroscience. She received a master degree in Biology at University of Naples and immediately after a PhD in Neuroscience. During her PhD she specialized in Neurogenetic aiming to identify new gene or new mutation in neurodegenerative disease. Then she moved in Belgium for a post doc and she specialized in molecular neuroscience, studying molecular mechanism of Fragile X Syndrome. She then returned back to Italy where she improved her career and expertise within behavioural field. Thanks to her expertise she is able to deeply analyze different aspects of neuroscience field. She participated in different international meetings and collaborated with group in Rome but also Milan, USA, etc. Actually her research is focused on the molecular mechanism of APP expression in normal and pathological condition in AD mice model (Tg2576). In particular, she analyzed the role of RNA Binding Protein (RBPs) in the APP metabolism and their regulation in APP expression, since APP is found overexpressed in AD patient with Swedish mutation (Johnston et al., 1994) but also in sporadic cases (Vignini et al., 2014; Borreca et al., 2015).

She has also observed an unbalance of two specific RBPs in the AD mice model and synaptosomes of AD sporadic patient: hnRNP C and FMRP (Borreca et al., 2015). She focused the research on the role of the protein synthesis machinery in the Alzheimer disease. In particular she analyzed the protein synthesis in the early phase of the pathology and distribution of APP mRNA on polysome fractionation as well as the role of some protein synthesis molecule in the Alzheimer pathology.

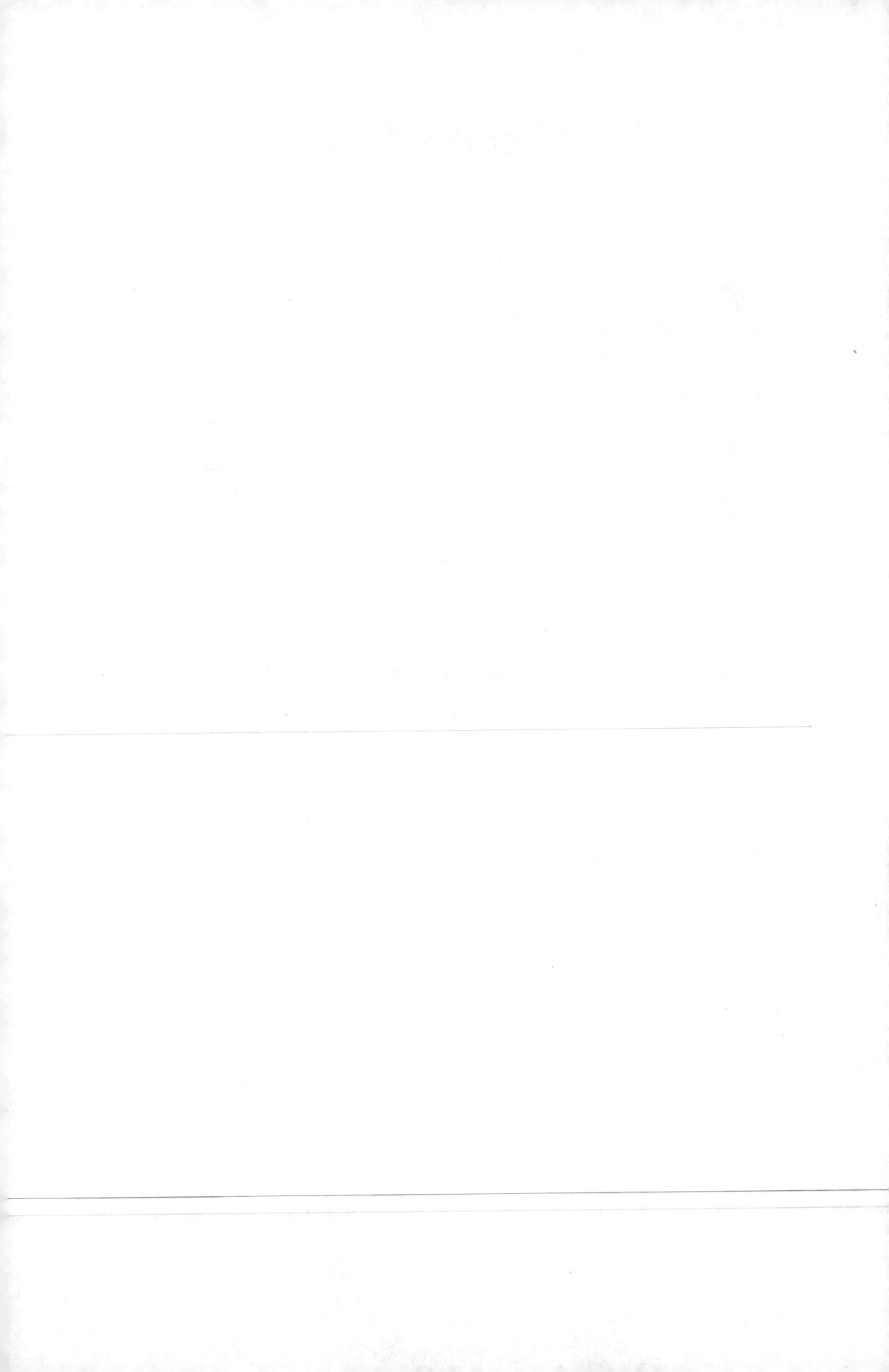

Contents

Preface

This Edited Volume is a collection of reviewed and relevant research chapters, concerning the developments within the neurodegeneration field of study. The book includes scholarly contributions by various authors and edited by a group of experts pertinent to neurodegeneration. Each contribution comes as a separate chapter complete in itself but directly related to the book's topics and objectives.

The book is divided in 5 chapters: 1. Introductory Chapter: A Common Feature of Neurodegenerative Disorders, 2. Neuroprotective Strategies of Blood-Brain Barrier Penetrant "Forskolin" (AC/cAMP/PK$_A$/CREB Activator) to Ameliorate Mitochondrial Dysfunctioning in Neurotoxic Experimental Model of Autism, 3. From Neuronal Differentiation of iPSCs to 3D Neural Organoids: Modeling of Neurodegenerative Diseases, 4. Molecular Basis of Neurodegeneration: Lessons from Alzheimer's and Parkinson's Diseases and 5. Neurodegenerative Diseases Associated with Mutations in SLC25A46.

The target audience comprises scholars and specialists in the field.

Antonella Borreca
Umberto Veronesi Post Doc Fellowship at Humanitas Research Hospital
Rome, Italy

Chapter 1

Introductory Chapter: A Common Feature of Neurodegenerative Disorders

Antonella Borreca

Additional information is available at the end of the chapter

http://dx.doi.org/10.5772/intechopen.84132

1. Introduction

The neurodegeneration is a common feature of different disorders, and many partners are involved in this mechanism. The last effect of degeneration is normally observed in the spine defects: reduction of spine density and alteration of morphology or functionality. The degeneration of neuron activity normally leads to the complete cell death.

The most neurodegenerative disorders are essentially affected by neurodegeneration of spine density and functionality, but the initial step or the trigger point is different from each other. Neurodevelopmental disorders or neurodegenerative disease related to the age affects patients in different ways but with the same effect. For this reason, a neurodegeneration is normally an intriguing topic for all scientific communities. Some of the molecular pathways involved in neurodegeneration associated to the most common neurodegenerative disorders are listed below.

2. Accumulation of protein

The aggregation of protein is normally considered a common feature of neurodegeneration. This accumulation leads to neurotoxicity and neuronal death. The causes of protein accumulation are different, but normally most of them are essentially due to mutation of regulation regions of gene (5′UTR, 3′UTR, etc.). Epigenetic mechanism occurs in regulation of protein synthesis, and accumulation of aggregated protein is a consequence Mus L et al., 2019; Sorrentino za et al 2019; Joppe K et al., 2019.

IntechOpen

3. Axonal degeneration

Communication from cell bodies to the peripheral spines happens due to the neuronal axon. Various insults may compromise this communication and deteriorate the neuronal axons: trauma, blockade of neuronal transport, or chemical toxicity. The normal trauma associated to axonal degeneration is nerve injury or some stroke. Protein involved in axonal transport deficit or accumulation of protein may also contribute to the axonal degeneration Correale et al., 2019.

4. Mitochondria dysfunction

Mitochondria are important organelles for cells, regulating the cell homeostasis. These organelles contribute to the cell energy, and alteration of one of their function may affect cell life.

Normally, brain senescence and neurodegeneration occur with mitochondrial dysfunction by impaired electron transfer and oxidative damage Cowan K et al., 2019.

5. Apoptosis alteration

Apoptotic cell pathway is a defense mechanism for neurons. Alteration of this system-induced neuronal loss in developing brain affects normal function of neuronal cells, leading to neurodegeneration.

DNA damage is also a common feature of apoptotic pathway, but when this pathway is altered, neuronal defect occurs and, as a consequence, neurodegenerative cell profile D'amelio et al, 2011.

6. Protein synthesis

Some mRNA are transferred locally at synapses and translated upon stimuli, when the protein is necessary. The alteration of global protein synthesis machinery locally at synapses is an important scenario of neurodegeneration and the main cause of different neurodevelopmental disorders Wong yl et al., 2019.

7. Alteration of receptor functionality

The neurons communicate with other neuronal cells through neurotransmitters. The neurotransmitters are released from presynaptic boutons to the postsynaptic compartments which are recognized by receptor. The neuronal receptors are classified as inhibitory and excitatory, and for this reason different effects are observed in neuron functionality. Mutation or alteration of neurotransmitters affects receptor functionality and neurodegenerative effect.

8. microRNA

Epigenetic mechanism affects cell activity and functionality. Recently, some papers demonstrate a functional role of microRNA in regulation of gene expression. The alteration of microRNA machinery alters gene expression and affects neuronal function Dardiotis E et al., 2018; wang xh et al., 2018.

9. Probably microglia and inflammation

Activation of inflammatory pathway generates a neuronal cascade molecule activation following the external stimuli. The inflammatory pathway is also responsible of synaptic pruning with the elimination of immature and nonactive spines. When this system is altered, many of neuronal activities are affected and neurodegeneration occurs.

The study of different molecular pathways of synaptic plasticity is one of the most intriguing mechanism to identify how neuronal works and intervene in neurodegenerative cases. Most of the neuronal diseases are linked to the neurodegeneration. For this reason, the study of this mechanism is essentially important in the field of neuroscience and is necessary to intervene in case of pathology Paasila pj et al., 2019.

Author details

Antonella Borreca

Address all correspondence to: antonella.borreca@gmail.com

CNR-National Research Council, Institute of Cell Biology and Neurobiology, Italy

Neuroprotective Strategies of Blood-Brain Barrier Penetrant "Forskolin" (AC/cAMP/PK$_A$/CREB Activator) to Ameliorate Mitochondrial Dysfunctioning in Neurotoxic Experimental Model of Autism

Sidharth Mehan, Himanshi Khera and Ramit Sharma

Additional information is available at the end of the chapter

http://dx.doi.org/10.5772/intechopen.80046

Abstract

New developments in the study of brain are among the most exciting frontiers of contemporary neuroscientific research for the clinical practitioner. Increasing knowledge of neurocomplications and of their discrete localization in the various regions of brain permits new modes of pharmacological management of some major neurological disorders like autism. The research work reported in this scheme is undertaken with an objective to explore the potential molecular targets (AC/cAMP/PK$_A$/CREB) for the development of newer therapeutics strategies (forskolin) for the management of neurological disorders and associated symptoms. Studies aimed at addressing these questions have fallen into two main categories: in-vivo behavioral paradigms and in-vitro differentiation biochemical, morphological and histopathological analysis. Therefore, first time, we aim to gather the propensity of mitochondrial cofactors, neuropathological mechanisms and various diagnostic methods to explore the clinical therapeutic strategies to ameliorate the neurodevelopmental disorder autism.

Keywords: neurodegeneration, autism, mitochondrial dysfunction, adenylyl cyclase, forskolin

1. Introduction

Neurological disorders are a heterogeneous group of diseases of the nervous system having different etiologies. They represent illnesses of the selective regions of the brain and nervous tissues which control vital physiological functions such as learning and memory, posture and coordination of movements of nerves/muscles [1]. A variety of CNS disorders including Alzheimer's disease (AD), Parkinson's disease, Huntington's disease, amyotrophic lateral sclerosis (ALS), autism spectrum disorders, brain abscess, multiple sclerosis, spinal cord injury, and cerebral stroke, traumatic brain injury are characterized primarily by neurodegeneration and neuroinflammation [2].

Intracellular molecules also known as secondary messengers such as cyclic nucleotides i.e. cAMP and cGMP play a critical role in neuronal signaling and synaptic plasticity by activation of several pathways like cAMP/PKA/CREB, cGMP/PKG/CREB and factors like brain-derived neurotrophic factor (BDNF) [3], semaphorins [4], netrin-1&16 [5], nerve growth factor (NGF) [6], Neurotrophins 3,4,5-inhibitory factors associated with myelin and myelin associated gly-coprotein [MAG] [7]. These pathways and factors are well known to help in neuronal survival, neurogenesis and protect neurons from injury [8].

Elevation of cAMP causes both short- and long-term increase in synaptic strength [9] and stimulates cholinergic neuronal cells to release acetylcholine [10]. But, the levels of cAMP and cGMP are reported to be decreased in neuropathological conditions including cerebral stroke and AD [11].

It has been reported that cerebral ischemia-induced energy failure also leads to reduction in the levels of key signaling molecules such as cAMP and cGMP and results in disruption of cAMP/PKA/CREB [11] and cGMP/PKG/CREB signaling pathways [12]. On the other hand it had been reported to impair hippocampal long-term potentiation (LTP), a neurophysiological correlate of memory [13], by inhibiting the activation of both cAMP/PKA/CREB [14] as well as cGMP/PKG/CREB pathways in ICH pathology [15]. The pyramidal CA1 neurons of hippo-campus, involved in learning and memory become vulnerable target in cerebral stroke [16]. Further, cAMP or cGMP dependent CREB phosphorylation has too been reported to induce long term memory (LTP) [17] and inhibit apoptotic and necrotic cell death [18].

CREB is a transcriptional factor responsible for synthesis of proteins which are important for the growth and development of synaptic connections and increase in synaptic strength [19]. Thus, agents that enhance cAMP/PKA/CREB &cGMP/PKG/CREB pathways have potential for the treatment of stroke [73], AD and other neurological diseases [20]. cAMP and cGMP mediate signaling of several neurotransmitters including serotonin, acetylcholine, glutamate and dopamine, which play important role in cognitive functioning [21]. The activation of the cAMP-dependent protein kinase [PKA] significantly inhibits TNF-α [22] and inducible nitric oxide synthase [iNOS] in astrocytes and macrophages [23] which are implicated in neuroinflammation [22] and oxidative stress, respectively [24]. cAMP system is closely involved in the regulation of BDNF expression too [25] which play important role in neuro-nal survival [3], synaptic plasticity [26], learning and memory [27]. Further elevation of cAMP and cGMP levels is known to restore the energy levels [28], reduce excitotoxic damage [29], prevent Aβ-mediated neurotoxicity [14], enhance biosynthesis and release of neuro-transmitters [22], inhibit apoptotic and necrotic cell death [30] leading to improvement in cognitive functioning [31]. Central administration of cAMP and cGMP has been reported to enhance neuronal survival [32] and memory performance [31]. In view of the above, the enhancement and prolongation of cAMP and cGMP signaling can thus be helpful in dealing with neurodegenerative disorders including ICH. This can be accomplished by activating the adenylyl cyclase enzyme, which metabolizes these cyclic nucleotides. Forskolin a major diterpenoid isolated from the roots of *Coleus forskohlii* directly activates the enzyme adenylyl cyclase, thereby increasing the intracellular level of cAMP and leading to various physiological effects.

Despite substantial research into neuroprotection, treatment options are still limited to supportive care and the management of complications. Currently available drugs provide symptomatic relief but do not stop progression of disease. Thus, the development of new therapeutic strategies remains an unmet medical need. Failure of current drug therapy may be due to their action at only one of the many neurotransmitters involved [33] or their inability to up regulate signaling messengers reported to have important role in neuronal excitability [34], neurotransmitter biosynthesis and release [35], neuronal growth and differentiation [30], synaptic plasticity and cognitive functioning [36].

2. Experimental animal model of PPA-induced neurotoxicity

Administration of PPA to rodents, results in CNS lesions that selectively target right lateral ventricle associated within striatum, cortex, cerebellum, hippocampus, amygdala recapitulating the regional and neuronal specificity of pathologic events especially in autism [37]. The mitochondrial toxin PPA interferes with the conversion of succinate to fumarate in TCA cycle, responsible for the generation of FADH$_2$ utilized in the complex-II in mitochondrial electron transport chain (ETC) by which it direct inhibits the activity of the mitochondrial metabolic enzyme succinate dehydrogenase and reduced the definite amount of NADH where it consumed in complex-I with the help of an enzyme complex-I (NADPH oxidase) as well as involve in the dysregulation of complex-IV (cytochrome c oxidase), is the final protein complex in the ETC helping to establish a transmembrane difference of proton electrochemical potential that the complex-V (ATP synthase) then uses to synthesize ATP [38].PPA has now become an experimental tool to study neuronal susceptibility and motor phenotypes that are characteristic of autism (**Figure 1**) [39].

In rats, PPA-induced lesions in brain region that are associated with elevated lactate levels resulted in increased NMDA-receptor binding. PPA toxicity arises from secondary excitotoxic mechanisms, whereby energy depletion within vulnerable neurons facilitates abnormal activation of NMDA receptors and subsequent Ca2+ influx [40]. Stimulating energy generation by administering creatine markedly attenuates PPA toxicity and ameliorates lesion volume, lactate production and ATP depletion in PPA-treated rats [41]. Numerous reports assert that PPA toxicity is associated with increased oxidative damage within the CNS. The involvement of impairments in intrinsic anti-oxidant protection pathways after PPA administration is further supported by observations of reduced glutathione (GSH) levels in autistic brain [42].

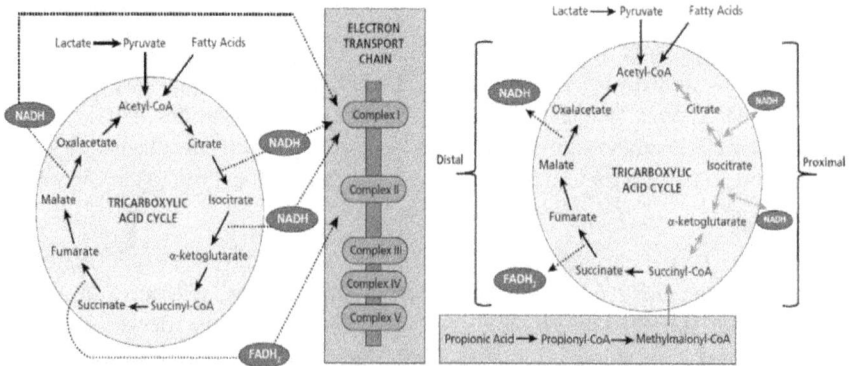

Figure 1. PPA-induced neurotoxicity; selective mitochondrial inhibition.

2.1. Propionic acid and autism

Propionic acid (PPA) is a short chain fatty acid formed endogenously in the human body as an intermediate of fatty acid metabolism and a metabolic end product of enteric gut micro biota such as clostridia and propionic bacteria [43–46]. MacFabe et al. and Shultz et al. have demonstrated that PPA intraventricularly infused to rats provides a suitable animal model to study autism. Being a weak organic acid, PPA exists in ionized and nonionized forms at physiological pH allowing it to readily cross lipid membranes, including the gut-blood and blood-brain barriers. PPA and other short-chain fatty acids (i.e., butyrate and acetate), affect diverse physiological processes such as cell signaling, neurotransmitter synthesis and release, mitochondrial

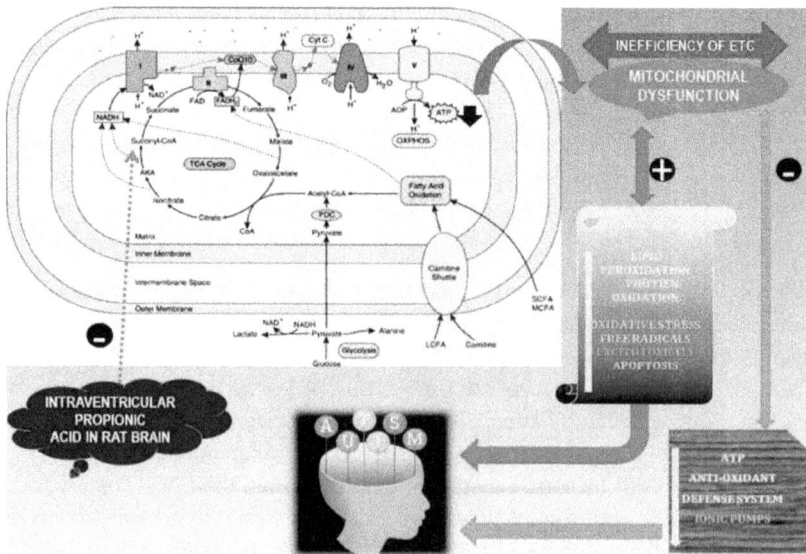

Figure 2. Intraventricular injection of PPA-inducing neurotoxic effect in mitochondrial respiratory chain (ETC).

function, lipid metabolism, immune functions, gap junctional gating, and modulation of gene expression through DNA methylation and histone acetylation [47]. Initial studies using this rodent model revealed that repeated brief infusions of PPA into the lateral cerebral ventricles (i.e., AP 1.3 mm, ML 1.8 mm, and DV 3.0 mm) of adult rats produced behavioral, biochemical, electrophysiological and neuropathological effects consistent with those seen in autism [43]. PPA through oxidative mechanisms inhibits Na+/K+ ATPase and increases glutamate receptor sensitivity which can enhance neural depolarization leading to neural hyper excitability in brain regions linked to locomotor activity (**Figure 2**).

Mitochondrial dysfunction has been well established to occur and play an important role in the pathogenesis of autism [48]. Preliminary magnetic resonance spectroscopy studies showed decreased synthesis of ATP and a disturbance of energy metabolism in the brain of individuals with autism. PPA is also capable of altering dopamine, serotonin, GABA and glutamate systems in a manner similar to that observed in autism [49].

3. List of proposed parameters can be evaluated on the basis of behavioral and biochemical alterations in neurotoxic experimental animal models of autism

Proposed experimental design of propionic acid-induced behavioral and biochemical estimations (**Figure 3**)

1. Measurement of body weight

2. Measurement of brain weight

3. Behavioral parameters

Spatial navigation task in Morris water maze, spontaneous locomotor activity, string test for grip strength, elevated plus maze test, beam crossing task, force swim test, rota rod apparatus

4. Estimation of biochemical parameters

Preparation of homogenate, estimation of biochemical parameters in serum and tissue homogenate such as protein estimation, lactate dehydrogenase (LDH) assay, estimation of malondialdehyde (MDA) levels, glutathione levels, superoxide dismutase (SOD) activity, catalase activity, acetyl cholinesterase (AChE) levels, determination of protein carbonyl (PC), nitrite levels

5. Estimation of biochemical parameters in serum and urine

Estimation of total urea, estimation of uric acid, estimation of biochemical parameters in tissue homogenate for mitochondrial complex activity

6. Preparation of crude mitochondrial fraction from rat whole brain homogenate

Complex-1 activity (NADPH dehydrogenase), complex-II activity (succinate dehydrogenase/SDH), complex IV activity (cytochrome oxidase), complex-V activity (ATP synthase)

7. Estimation of biochemical parameters in serum

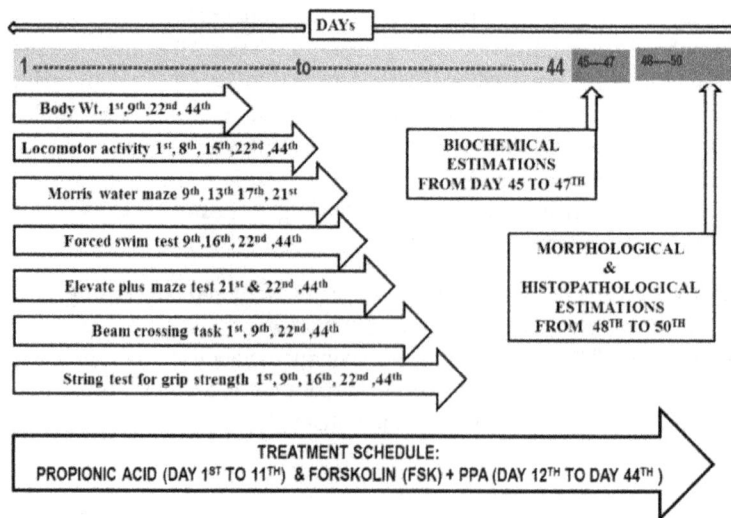

Figure 3. Proposed experimental design: propionic acid-induced behavioral and biochemical estimations.

Estimation of complete blood count (CBC) such as determination of different hematological parameters, such as red blood cells (RBC), white blood cells (WBCs), hemoglobin (HB), hematocrit (HCT), mean corpuscular volume (MCV), mean corpuscular hemoglobin (MCH), mean corpuscular hemoglobin concentration (MCHC), red blood cell distribution width (RDW), neutrophils%, lymphocytes%, monocytes%, eosinophil's%, basophils%, mean platelet volume (MPV), platelet distribution width (PDW)%, plateletcrit (PCT)% and platelets (PLTs) was measured in rat serum or blood sample

8. Miscellaneous

Estimation of blood glucose levels, triglycerides levels, total cholesterol levels, serum C-reactive protein (CRP) levels

9. Inflammatory parameters in tissue homogenate-enzyme-linked immunosorbent assay (ELISA)

Estimation of TNF-α, interleukin-1β (IL-1β), interleukin-6 (IL-6), interleukin-10 (IL-10)

10. Estimation of biochemical parameters in urine

Urine output, urine dipstick test

11. Histopathological and morphological sections studies

12. Immunohistochemistry

4. Future perspectives and treatment approach

Phytochemicals drugs have been used since ancient times as medicines for treatment of a range of diseases. Medicinal plants have played a key role in world health. In spite of the great advances observed in modern medicine in recent decades, plants still make an important contribution to health care. Medicinal plants are distributed worldwide, but they are most abundant in tropical countries. Over the past decade, interest in drugs derived from higher plants, especially the phototherapeutic ones, has increased expressively. It is estimated that about 25% of all modern medicines are directly or indirectly derived from higher plants. Phytomedicines are standardized herbal preparation consisting of complex mixtures of one or more plants which are used in most countries for the management of various diseases. Other characteristics of phytochemicals are their wide therapeutic use and great acceptance by the population. In contrast to modern medicines, phytochemicals are frequently used to treat chronic diseases. Phytochemicals are normally marketed as standardized preparations in the form of liquid, solid, or various preparations. Compared with well-defined synthetic drugs, phytochemicals exhibit some marked differences, namely:

- The empirical use in folk medicine is a very important characteristic.

- They have a wide range of therapeutic use and are suitable for chronic treatments.

- The occurrence of undesirable side effects seems to be less frequent with herbal medicines, but well-controlled randomized clinical trials have revealed that they also exist.

- They usually cost less than synthetic drugs

5. Forskolin (*Coleus forskohlii*)

Coleus forskohlii known as phashana bedi (Telugu) a medicinal plant found in the Indian subcontinent is widely used in the Indian system of medicine. Forskolin (FSK) (also known as Colonels) is labdane diterpene that is obtained from the tuberous roots of *Coleus forskohlii*, which belongs to the family of Lamiaceae. *Coleus Forskohlii* is one of the world's most researched plant in which FSK is believed to be the plant's most active constituent. *C. forskohlii* has been used as an important folk medicine in India. *C. forskohlii* is a perennial herb and grows wild in arid and semi-arid regions of India, Nepal and Thailand; the roots have long been used in Ayurvedic medicine [50]. In traditional medicine, *C. forskohlii* is commonly used in different countries for various health disorders including cardiovascular diseases, hypertension, asthma, glaucoma and Alzheimer's disease. Its further use in promoting lean body mass, treating mood disorders and its anticancer activities is well known.

6. Medicinal properties of forskolin

Traditionally, the roots have been used as condiments in pickles, for preparation of pickles. Forskolin has positive effect against a wide range of conditions such as asthma, glaucoma, hypertension, hair loss, cancer, and obesity [51]. *C. forskohlii* extract (standardized to contain 95% forskolin) is potentially useful in skin care formulations, particularly as a conditioning age. In traditional Indian systems of medicine, the roots of *C. forskohlii* are used as a tonic. Other therapeutically relevant properties include anthelmintic action and efficacy in the management of skin infections and eruptions. The plant is also used traditionally in veterinary practice (**Table 1**). Essential oil in tubers of this plant has potential uses in food flavoring industry and can be used as an antimicrobial agent and has very attractive and delicate odor with spicy note. A labdane diterpenoid is considered the active secondary metabolite because of its ability to activate the enzyme adenylyl cyclase (Ac) thereby increasing the intracellular level of cAMP and leading to various physiological effects [52]. FSK is shown to exert a 6–400 fold increase in levels of cAMP. Cyclic AMP is a "second messenger" hormone signaling system as its synthesis triggers the action of various hormones, enzymes and other biological activities that have profound effects on local cells, as well as systemic effects, in some instances, on the entire body [53]. FSK by passes the adrenoreceptors, increasing cAMP levels directly, thereby stimulating lipolysis. FSK has also been shown to counteract the decreased response of fat cells to epinephrine, associated with aging. FSK also accelerates lipolysis through the activation of hormone-sensitive lipase [54]. It is primarily via the increased synthesis of cyclic AMP that *C. Forskohlii* may exert its medicinal influences on a significant number of common health conditions.

S.No.	Pharmacological activity	Mechanism of action	Ref. No
i.	Anti-depressant	FSK stimulated AC activity in rat brain and leads to enhancement of the coupling between stimulatory GTP-binding protein (G protein) and AC catalytic molecules FSK stimulates AC and regulates brain-derived neurotrophic factor (BDNF) and TrkB expression in the rat brain	92
ii.	Anti-Alzheimer's	FSK-induced abipolar neuron-like cell morphology and it enables neurogenin-2 (Ngn2) to convert human fibroblasts into cholinergic neurons Neuronal differentiation of adult rat neural progenitor cells (NCP's) was achieved	93
iii.	Anti-cancer	Restoration of PP2A activity with forskolin that inhibit Akt and ERK activity and block proliferation and induce caspase-dependent apoptosis in AML cell lines. Forskolin inhibited the *in-vivo* leukemogenesis of imatinib sensitive and resistant BCR/ABL+ 32Dcl3 cells in mice	94
iv.	Antispasmodic activity	increase of cAMP inhibit cramping or smooth muscle contraction	95
v.	Anti-Glaucoma	Stimulates Adenylate cyclase which stimulates the ciliary epithelium to produce cyclic adenosine monophosphate (cAMP) that results in decreased aqueous humor inflow there by decrease in IOP Reduction of intra ocular pressure	96
vi.	Cardioprotective amelioration of Mitochondrial dysfunction in cardiomyopathy	It reduces diastolic blood pressure without increasing myocardial oxygen consumption. Reduction of I_{Na} (cardiac Na + current) and overproduction of mitochondrial ROS in deoxycorticosterone acetate (DOCA) mouse myocytes by activating PKA and PKC	97
vii.	Anti-asthmatic	Forskolin activation of cAMP inhibits human basophil and mast cell degranulation, resulting in subsequent bronchodilation	98

S.No.	Pharmacological activity	Mechanism of action	Ref. No
viii.	Anti-psoriasis	Decreased cGMP levels that are associated with cell proliferation and thus decrease cell division. Normalizing the cAMP /cGMP ratio	99
ix.	Hepatoprotective activity	Repair of hepatic tissue damage, normalization of inflammatory hepatic and necrosis Forskolin increases cAMP accumulation, and therefore stimulates lipolysis.	100
x.	Anti-inflammatory	Reduction in the level of Interleukin-1β, 6 and 8 Overexpression of TANK-binding kinase 1 (TBK1) reduced phosphorylation of hormone-sensitive lipase (HSL) in response to FSK Inhibit mast cell degranulation	101
xi.	Anti-diabetic activity	FSK predominantly decreased basal glucose in healthy rats and attenuated the severity of hyperglycemia in diabetic rats FSK increase intracellular cAMP, which, together with the increase in ATP, enhance the priming of insulin granules	102
xii.	Anti-platelet aggregation	Antagonizes the action of platelet-activating factor (PAF). Reduction in the extent of platelet aggregation Induced a partial deaggregation of ADP- or collagen-aggregated human platelets	103
xiii.	Inhibition of human neutrophil degranulation Anti-histaminic activity	cAMP-mediated phosphodiesterase inhibition. Reduction in the histamine release from human basophiles and mast cells by modulating the release of mediators of the immediate hypersensitivity reaction, through activation of AC	104
xiv.	Smooth muscle relaxant	Increase both the cytosolic Ca^{2+} concentration and the cytosolic NO concentration ([NO]c) in the endothelial cells leads to cause vasodilatation Increases uterine smooth muscle AC	105
xv.	Hydrodynamic alterations in collecting tubule Anti-cystic fibrosis	FSK resulted in increase in osmotic water flux and hydraulic conductivity of the rabbit cortical collecting tubule FSK leads to cyst formation in culture media	106

Table 1. Pharmacological action of FSK.

7. FSK and brain

7.1. FSK-binding sites

3H-forskolin has, for example, been found to bind to both a high and a low affinity site in rat brain membranes [55] and the capacity of the high affinity forskolin-binding site has been shown to be increased by the activation of N-proteins by guanine nucleotides [56]. High affinity [3H] FSK-binding sites have been mapped autoradiographically in rat brain area such as caudate-putamen, nucleus accumbens, olfactory tubercle, globus pallidus, substantia nigra and the hilus of the area dentata [57] and exhibit a markedly heterogeneous distribution.

7.2. Role of FSK in brain

FSK may activate Ac by interacting with two sites, one which may be directly located on the cyclase molecule, and the other which is associated with OJ somehow formed by the interactions with the N, protein. FSK, a commonly used activator of Ac [55], elevates the stimulation-induced release of several transmitters, such as acetylcholine, noradrenaline and 5-hydrdoxytryptamine, from brain or synaptosomes and markedly increasing the rate of conversion of ATP to cyclic AMP [58]. FSK directly reduces certain K + −potassium currents in addition to its action on Ac. cAMP could increase the apparent number of Na, K-ATPase sites by either direct or indirect mechanisms. cAMP could increase the number of Na, K-ATPase sites by increasing cell Na + or decreasing K + though there are reports of Na, K-ATPase stimulation that may be independent of cation changes. FSK elevates electrically evoked acetylcholine release in the hippocampus independently of Ac activation [58]. FSK appears to provide a new clue for elucidating the physiological role of cAMP in the synaptic transmission in the sympathetic ganglia. FSK exerts two opposite pharmacological actions at the synapse, i.e. a facilitation of transmitter release at the presynaptic site and a depressant action on nicotinic acetylcholine receptor at the postsynaptic site. FSK reduced the amplitude shock stimulation of preganglionic nerve. FSK induces a reversible AChR desensitization at the junctional and extrajunctional regions in rat [59]. FSK, an activator of Ac, could increase transmitter release presynaptically in CA1 neurons. FSK directly stimulates Ac and thereby increases cyclic AMP activity, which is known to influence neurite outgrowth and membrane trafficking in neurons. Increased cyclic AMP activity may have multiple effects on cells including changing the direction of growing neurites [60] and increasing the density of clathrin-coated pits and coated vesicles at plasma membranes coincident with an increased synthesis of clathrin light chain. The cAMP effector system enhanced by FSK is involved in the release of dopamine from dopaminergic nerve endings in the neostriatum [61]. FSK increased dopamine formation in rat striatal slices, rat striatal synaptosomes, rat hypothalamic synaptosomes and bovine retinal slices [62].

8. Neuroprotective action of FSK

8.1. FSK against neuroinflammation

An increase in intracellular cAMP levels through FSK to play an important role in modulating the cytokine production. Intracellular cAMP has been reported to depress the accumulation of tumor necrosis factor (TNF-α) an mRNA by inhibiting the transcriptional processes. Elevation of intracellular cAMP levels induced by PDE inhibitors, FSK, prostaglandin E2, or cell-permeable cAMP analogue also inhibited the secretion of IL-1b, whereas it increased IL-1b mRNA levels from lipopolysaccharide-stimulated human monocytes. Although the regulatory modality of IL-8 production by cAMP is still unclear and depends on the cell type, enhanced cAMP appears to have favorable effects at least on airway cells by suppressing IL-8 production [63]. Therefore, enhanced cAMP levels by have also FSK been recognized to reverse the increased pulmonary microvascular permeability associated with ischemia reperfusion (**Figure 4**) [64].

8.2. Forskolin against neurooxidation

Oxidative stress may play a role in the development and clinical manifestations of autism. Both central and peripheral markers of oxidative stress have been reported in autism. Peripheral markers have included lipid peroxidation levels. Increases in these markers correlated with loss of previously acquired language skills in autism. Furthermore, metabolic markers of oxidative stress have been identified including abnormal levels of metabolites signifying impaired methylation and increased oxidative stress in autism [65]. The oxidative stress in autism may be caused by an imbalance between the generation of ROS and the defense mechanism against ROS by antioxidants. An increase in reactive oxygen species (ROS) results in damage to proteins, DNA, and lipids. Specifically, the interaction between ROS and nitric oxide (NO) results in the nitration of tyrosine residues in proteins and can alter protein conformation and function [66]. Oxidative DNA damage is also considered to play an important role in the pathology of a number of diseases like Parkinson's disease, tardive dyskinesia, metal intoxication syndromes, Down's syndrome, and possibly also in schizophrenia, Huntington's disease, and Alzheimer's disease. Reactive oxygen species including superoxide ($O2.-$), hydroxyl ($.OH$), hydrogen peroxide (H_2O_2), singlet oxygen ($1O^2$) and nitric oxide ($NO\bullet$) can cause cellular injury when they are generated excessively or the enzymatic and nonenzymatic antioxidant defense systems are impaired [67].

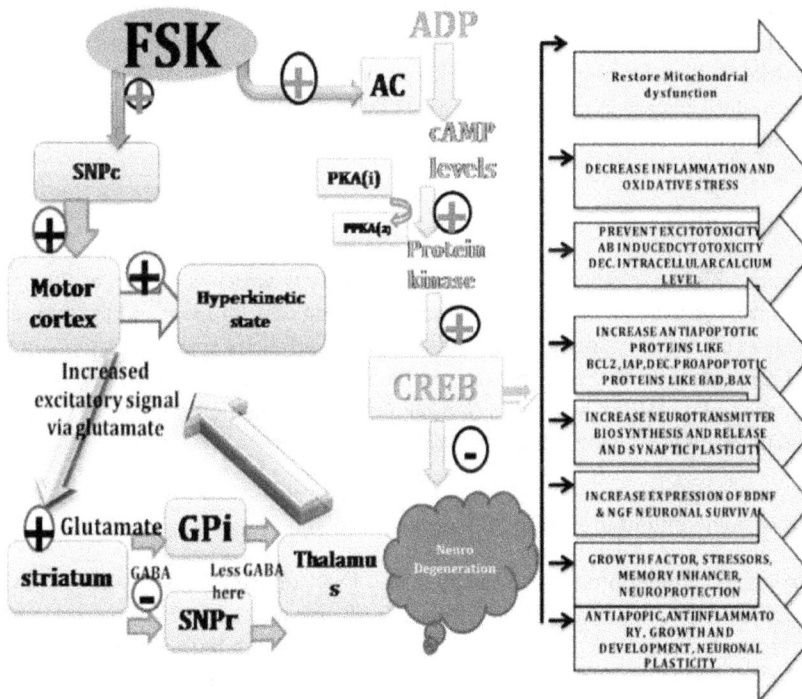

Figure 4. Neuroprotective action of forskolin-mediated AC/cAMP/PKA/CREB activation.

Moreover, FSK-mediated cAMP/PKA/CREB activation were found to inhibit LPS- and cytokine-mediated production of NO as well as the expression of iNOS, whereas compounds (H-89 and (Rp)-cAMP) that decrease PKA activity stimulated the production of NO and the expression of iNOS in rat primary astrocytes [68].

8.3. Forskolin against mitochondrial dysfunctioning

The brain is strongly dependent on the ATP production of the cell energy-producing organelle, the mitochondrion. There is a large body of evidence involving mitochondrial dysfunctions in ASD. Palmieri and Persico, regarding ASD, oxidative phosphorylation (OXPHOS) in the mitochondrion requires at least 80 proteins, of which only 13 are encoded by the mtDNA, while mitochondrial functioning has been estimated to need the participation of approximately 1500 nuclear genes. Mitochondrial dysfunction is present in the brains of individuals with ASD and may play a role in its core cognitive and behavioral symptoms. Alternatively, mitochondria can be damaged by endogenous stressors associated with ASD such as elevated pro-inflammatory cytokines resulting from an activated immune system or other conditions associated with oxidative stress. Oxidative stress may be a key link between mitochondrial dysfunction and ASD as reactive oxygen species (ROS) generated from pro-oxidant environmental toxicants and activated immune cells can result in mitochondrial dysfunction. Excess production of free radicals or impaired antioxidant mechanisms may cause oxidative stress: impaired mitochondrial function then leads to further oxidative stress and a vicious negative cycle can ensue. Instead, abnormal functioning appears secondary to excessive Ca2+ levels. Mitochondrial dysfunctioning caused depletion of ATP, that further decrease the level of cAMP. Forskolin, increase in intracellular cAMP, through the phosphorylation of CREB which perform neuroprotective functioning associate with mitochondrial dysfunctioning [69].

8.4. Forskolin against cognitive dysfunction

Autistic brain which may reflect enhanced cortical plasticity which is defined as the process of microstructural construction of synapses occurring during development and the remodeling of these synapses during learning [70]. Enhanced synaptic plasticity triggers a regional reorganization of brain functions that account for both the unique aspects of autism and its variability [71]. Activation of cAMP/PKA has been mainly implicated in stimulating learning and memory. FSK activate cAMP/CREB in hippocampal region [72].

8.5. Possible involvement of FSK in PPA-induced autism

Summarizing the whole information given above, FSK confirmed a versatile role in autism where it activates the AC/cAMP-mediated PK_A/CREB activation. Moreover, on other side FSK act as a co-activator in brain that follows the G_S pathway through the activation of D1 receptor. There is least availability of selective AC activation and so far only limited reports suggest beneficial effect of FSK in neurodegeneration animal model.

9. Conclusion

In conclusion, the current study strongly confirms that the administration of propionic acid induces brain lesions that are similar to the behavioral, histological, morphological, biochemical, neurochemical, and pathological features of autism. After Chronic administration of propionic acid in the rats as proven by motor dysfunctions, biochemical and neurochemical alternations. The literature finding in the current study reveals that adenylyl cyclase activator, that is, FSK-mediated cAMP/CREB activation, might be a unique platform for the prevention of neurodegenerative diseases. Thus in conclusion, neuroprotective and neuro restoration effects of FSK may be due to favorable modulation of CREB-mediated signaling. The involvement of cAMP/PK$_A$/CREB pathway, anti-oxidant, anti-inflammatory and neuroprotective effect of test drug FSK may be the possible mechanisms at least in part underlying the observed effects (**Figure 4**).

Furthermore, with cAMP/PK$_A$/CREB signaling in regulation of neuronal functioning, the future studies can be designed to investigate the protective and therapeutic potency of forskolin in animal models of brain hemorrhage, Huntington's disease and Parkinson's disease and to find out if cAMP-mediated CREB pathway is equally implicated in the disease pathogenesis or progression. So, now we can finally conclude the significant mitochondrial restorative effects of the FSK may be due to showing its improved motor and cognitive functions as well as to restore the energy levels and antioxidant and anti-inflammatory defense system.

Acknowledgements

The authors express their gratitude to Chairman, Mr. Parveen Garg, and Director, Dr. G.D. Gupta, ISF College of Pharmacy, Moga (Punjab), India, for their great vision and support. Authors are really thankful to Dr. Vikramdeep Monga, for valuable support and encouragement.

Author details

Sidharth Mehan*, Himanshi Khera and Ramit Sharma

*Address all correspondence to: sidh.mehan@gmail.com

Department of Pharmacology, ISF College of Pharmacy, Moga, Punjab, India

References

[1] Swerdlow RH. Mitochondrial DNA–related mitochondrial dysfunction in neurodegenerative diseases. Archives of Pathology & Laboratory Medicine. 2002;**126**:271-280

[2] Kermer P, Liman J, Jochen H. Neuronal apoptosis in neurodegenerative diseases: From basic research to clinical application. Neurodegenerative Diseases. 2004;1:9-19

[3] Song JH, Huang CS, Nagata K, Yeh JZ, Narahash T. Differential action of riluzole on tetrodotoxin-sensitive and tetrodotoxin-resistant sodium channels. Journal of Pharmacology and Experimental Therapeutics. 1997;282:707

[4] Chalasani SH, Sabelko KA, Sunshine MJ. A chemokine, SDF-1, reduces the effectiveness of multiple axonal repellents and is required for normal axon pathfinding. The Journal of Neuroscience. 2003;23:1360-1371

[5] Shewan D, Dwivedy A, Anderson R, Holt CE. Age-related changes underlie switch in netrin-1 responsiveness as growth cones advance along visual pathway. Nature Neuroscience. 2002;5(10):955-962

[6] Akassoglou K. Nerve growth factor-independent neuronal survival: A role for NO donors. Molecular Pharmacology. 2005;68(4):952-955

[7] Cai D, Qiu J, Cao Z. Neuronal cyclic AMP controls the developmental loss in ability of axons to regenerate. The Journal of Neuroscience. 2001;21(13):4731-4739

[8] Frey U, Huang YY, Kandel ER. Effects of cAMP simulates a late stage of LTP in hippocampal CA1 neurons. Science. 1993;260:1661-1664

[9] Marx G. The Molecular Basis of Memory. Acs Chemistry. Neuroscience. 2012;3:633-642

[10] Yao WD, Rusch J, Poo MM, Wu CF. Spontaneous acetylcholine secretion from developing growth cones of Drosophila central neurons in culture: Effects of cAMP-pathway mutations. The Journal of Neuroscience. 2000;20:2626-2637

[11] Nagakura A, Niimura M, Takeo S. Effects of a phosphodiesterase IV inhibitor rolipram on microsphere embolism-induced defects in memory function and cerebral cyclic AMP signal transduction system in rats. British Journal of Pharmacology. 2002;135:1783-1794

[12] Zhou X, Xiao-Wei D, Crona J. Vinpocetine is a potent blocker of rat $Na_V1.8$ TTX-resistant sodium channels. Journal of Pharmacology and Experimental Therapeutics. 2003;306:498-504

[13] Bliss TVP, Collingridge GL. A synaptic model of memory: Long-term potentiation in the hippocampus. Nature. 1993;361:31-39

[14] Vitolo OV, Angelo AS, Costanzo V. Amyloid beta-peptide inhibition of the PKA/CREB pathway and long-term potentiation: Reversibility by drugs that enhance cAMP signaling. Proceedings of the National Academy of Sciences. 2002;99:13217-13221

[15] Puzzo D, Vitolo O, Trinchese F. Neurobiology of disease amyloidβ peptide inhibits activation of the nitric oxide/cGMP/cAMP-responsive element-binding protein pathway during hippocampal synaptic plasticity. The Journal of Neuroscience. 2005;25:6887-6897

[16] Euler MV, Bendel O, Bueters T. Profound but transient deficits in learning and memory after global ischemia using novel water maze test. Behavioral Brain Research. 2006;166:204-210

[17] Hardingham GE, Arnold FJ, Bading H. Nuclear calcium signaling controls CREB-mediated gene expression triggered by synaptic activity. Nature Neuroscience. 2001;4: 261-267

[18] Francois M, Le Cabec V, Dupont MA. Induction of necrosis in human neutrophils by Shigellaflexneri requires type III secretion, IpaB and IpaCinvasins, and actin polymerization. Infection and Immunity. 2000;68:1289-1296

[19] Finkbeiner S. CREB couples neurotrophin signals to survival messages. Neuron. 2000;25: 11-14

[20] Gong B, Vitolo OV, Trinchese F. Persistent improvement in synaptic and cognitive functions in an Alzheimer mouse model after rolipram treatment. The Journal of Clinical Investigation. 2004;114:1624-1634

[21] Fujita M, Zoghbi TSS, Crescenzo MS. Quantification of brain phosphodiesterase 4 in rat with (R)-[11C]Rolipram-PET. Neuro Image. 2005;26:1201-1210

[22] Chong YH, Shin YJ, Suh YH. Cyclic AMP inhibition of tumor necrosis factor production induced by amuloidigenic c-terminal peptide of Alzheimer's amyloid precursor protein in macrophages: Involvement of multiple pathways and cyclic AMP response element binding protein. Molecular Pharmacology. 2003;63:690-698

[23] Pahan K, Namboodiri AMS, Sheikh FG. Increasing cAMP attenuates induction of inducible nitric-oxide synthase in rat primary astrocytes. The Journal of Biological Chemistry. 1997;272(12):7786-7791

[24] Nakamura Y. Regulating factors for microglial activation. Biological & Pharmaceutical Bulletin. 2002;25(8):945-953

[25] Zafra F, Lindholm D, Thoenen H. Regulation of brain-derived neurotrophic factor and nerve growth factor mRNA in primary cultures of hippocampal neurons and astrocytes. The Journal of Neuroscience. 1992;12:4793-4799

[26] Rutten K, Lieben C, Smits L. The PDE4 inhibitor rolipram reverses object memory impairment induced by acute tryptophan depletion in the rat. Psychopharmacology. 2007;192: 275-282

[27] Nibuya M, Nestler EJ, Duman RS. Chronic antidepressant administration increases the expression of cAMP response element binding protein (CREB) in rat hippocampus. The Journal of Neuroscience. 1996;16:2365-2372

[28] Flamm ES, Schiffer J, Viau AT. Alterations of cyclic AMP in cerebral ischemia. Stroke. 1978;9:400-402

[29] Yoshioka A, Shimizu Y, Hirose G. Cyclic AMP-elevating agents prevent oligodendroglial excitotoxicity. Journal of Neurochemistry. 1998;70:2416-2423

[30] Silveira MS, Linden R. Neuroprotection by cAMO: Another brick in the wall. In: Brain Repair. Advances in Experimental Medicine and Biology. 2006;557:164-176

[31] Rutten K, Prickaerts J, Hendrix M. Time-dependent involvement of cAMP and cGMP in consolidation of object memory: Studies using selective phosphodiesterase type 2, 4 and 5 inhibitors. European Journal of Pharmacology. 2007;**558**:107-112

[32] Prickaert J, Sik A, van Staveren WC, Koopmans G, Steinbusch HW, van der Staay FJ. Phosphodiesterase type 5 inhibition improves early memory consolidation of object information. Neurochemistry International. 2004;**45**:915-928

[33] Rose GM, Hopper A, De Vivo M, Tehim A. Phosphodiesterase inhibitors for cognitive enhancement. Current Pharmaceutical Design. 2005;**11**(26):3329-3334

[34] Bach ME, Barad M, Son H. Age-related defects in spatial memory are correlated with defectsin the late phase of hippocampal long-term potentiation in vitroand are attenuated by drugs that enhance the cAMP signaling pathway. Proceedings of the National Academy of Sciences. 1999;**96**:5280-5285

[35] Rutten K, Prickaerts J, Blokland A. Rolipram reverses scopolamine-induced and time-dependent memory deficits in object recognition by different mechanisms of action. Neurobiology of Learning and Memory. 2006;**85**:132-138

[36] Rydel RE, Greenet LA. cAMP analogs promote survival and neurite outgrowth in cultures of rat sympathetic and sensory neurons independently of nerve growth factor (neurotrophic agents/neuronal regeneration/neuronal differentiaion/8-(4-chlorophenylthio)-cAMP/8-bromo-cAMP). Proceedings of the National Academy of Sciences. 1998;**85**:1257-1261

[37] Xu Y, Liu P, Li Y. Impaired development of mitochondria plays a role in the central nervous system defects of fetal alcohol syndrome. Birth Defects Research Part A: Clinical and Molecular Teratology. 2005 Feb;**73**(2):83-91

[38] MacFabe D. Autism: Metabolism, mitochondria, and the microbiome. Global Advances in Health and Medicine. 2013;**6**:52-63

[39] Shultz SR, MacFabe DF. Intracerebroventricular injections of the enteric bacterial metabolic product propionic acid impair cognition and sensorimotor ability in the long-Evans rat: Further development of a rodent model of autism. Behavioural Brain Research. 2009;**200**:33-41

[40] Nakao S, Fujii A, Niederman R. Alteration of cytoplasmic Ca2+ in resting and stimulated human neutrophils by short-chain carboxylic acids at neutral pH. Infection and Immunity. 1992;**60**:5307-5311

[41] Thomas RH, Folley KA, Mepham JR, Tichenoff LJ, Posmeyer F, MacFabe DF. Altered brain phospholipid and acylcarnitine profiles in propionic acid infused rodents: Further development of a potential model of autism spectrum disorders. Journal of Neurochemistry. 2014;**113**:515-529

[42] Bloom FE. The role of cyclic nucleotides in central synaptic function. Reviews of Physiology, Biochemistry and Pharmacology. 1975;**74**:1-103

[43] Al-Gadani Y, El-Ansary A, Attas O, Al-Ayadhi L. Oxidative stress and antioxidant status in Saudi autistic children. Clinical Biochemistry. 2009;**42**:1032-1040

[44] Finegold SM, Dowd SE, Gontcharova V, Liu C, Henley KE, Wolcott RD. Pyrosequencing study of fecal microflora of autistic and control children. Anaerobe. 2010;**16**:444-453

[45] Paxinos G, Watson C. The Rat Brain in Stereotaxic Coordinates. Montreal: Academic Press; 1986

[46] Cummings JH, Pomare EW, Branch WJ, Naylor CP, Macfarlane GT. Short chain fatty acids in human large intestine, portal, hepatic and venous blood. Gut. 1987;**28**:1221-7.22

[47] Wagner CG, Reuhl KR, Cheh M, McRae P, Halladay AK. A new neurobehavioral model of autism in mice: Pre- and postnatal exposure to sodium valproate. Journal of Autism and Developmental Disorders. 2006;**36**:779-793

[48] Brock M, Buckel W. On the mechanism of action of the antifungal agent propionate. European Journal of Biochemistry. 2004;**271**:3227-3241

[49] Moran PM, Higgins LS, Cordell B, Moser PC. Age related learning deficts in transgenic mice expressing the 751-amino acid isoform of human beta amyloid precursor protein. Proceedings of the National Academy of Sciences of the United States of America. 1995; **92**(12):5341-5345

[50] Dubey MP, Srimal RC, Nityanand S, Dhawan BN. Pharmacological studies on coleonol, a hypertensive diterpene from *Coleus forskohlii*. Journal of Ethnopharmacology. 1981;**3**:1-13

[51] Ammon HP, Müller AB. Forskolin: From an ayurvedic remedy to a modern agent. Planta medica. 1985 Dec;**51**(06):473-477

[52] Seamon KB, Daly JW. Forskolin: Unique diterpene activator of adenylatecyclase in membranes and intact cells. Journal of Cyclic Nucleotide Research. 1981;**7**:201-224

[53] Abraham Z. In: Jain SK, editor. Glimpses of Indian Ethnobotany. Bombay: Oxford & IBM Publishing Co.; 1981. p. 315

[54] Allen DO. Relationships between cyclic AMP levels and lipolysis in fat cells after isoproterenol and forskolin stimulation. The Journal of Pharmacology and Experimental Therapeutics. 1986;**2**:659-664

[55] Li H, Yang W, Mendes F, Amaral MD, Sheppard DN. Impact of the cystic fibrosis mutation F508del-CFTR on renal cyst formation and growth. American Journal of Physiology. Renal Physiology. 2012;**303**:1176-1186

[56] Seamon KB. Forskolin and Adenylate Cyclase: New Opportunities in Drug Design. InAnnual reports in medicinal chemistry. Academic Press. 1984 Jan 1;**19**:293-302

[57] Seamon KB, Daly JW. High-affinity binding of forskolin to rat brain membranes. Advances in cyclic nucleotide and protein phosphorylation research. 1985;**19**:125-135

[58] Seamon KB, Daly JW. Forskolin: Its biological and chemical properties. Advances in Cyclic Nucleotide and Protein Phosphorylation Research. 1986;**20**:1-150

[59] Worley PF, Baraban JM, Snyderi SH. Lnositol 1,4,5-trisphosphate receptor binding: Autoradiographic localization in rat brain. The Journal of Neuroscience. 1989;**l**:339-348

[60] Allgaier C, Choi BK, Hertting G. Forskolin modulates acetylcholine release in the hippocampus independently of adenylatecyclase activation. European Journal of Pharmacology. 1990;**181**:279-282

[61] Albuquerque EX, Deshpande SS, Aracava Y, Alkondon M, Daly D. A possible involvement of cyclic AMP in the expression of desensitization of the nicotinic acetylcholine receptor. 1986;**199**:1-8

[62] Song HJ, Ming GI, Poo MM. cAMP-induced switching in turning direction of nerve growth cones. Nature. 1997;**388**:275-279

[63] Hu Y, Barzilai A, Chen M, Bailey CH, Kandel ER. 5-HT and cAMP induce the formation of coated pits and vesicles and increase the expression of clathrin light chain in sensory neurons of aplysia. Neuron. 1993;**10**:921-929

[64] Bailly S, Ferrua B, Fay M, Gougerot-Pocidalo MA. Differential regulation of IL 6, IL 1A, IL 1b and TNFa production in LPS-stimulated human monocytes: Role of cyclic AMP. Cytokine. 1990;**2**:205-210

[65] Zitnik RJ, Zheng T, Elias JA. CAMP inhibition of interleukin-1–induced interleukin-6 production by human lung fibroblasts. The American Journal of Physiology. 1993;**264**(3): L253-L260

[66] Tang L, Okamoto S, Shiuchi T. Sympathetic nerve activity maintains an antiinflammatory state in adipose tissue in male mice by inhibiting TNF-gene expression in macrophages. Endocrinology. 2015:1-14

[67] Meguid NA, Dardir AA, Abdel-Raouf ER, Hashish A. Evaluation of oxidative stress in autism: Defective antioxidant enzymes and increased lipid peroxidation. Biological Trace Element Research. 2011;**143**:58-65

[68] Elizabeth M, Sajdel-Sulkowska, Xu M, Koibuchi N. Increase in cerebellar Neurotrophin-3 and oxidative stress markers in autism. Cerebellum. 2009;**8**:366-372

[69] Arnould T, Vankoningsloo S, Renard P. CREB activation induced by mitochondrial dysfunctions is anew signaling pathway that impairs cell proliferation. The EMBO Journal. 2002;**22**(1&2):53-63

[70] Kamata H, Tanaka C, Yagisawa H, Hirata H. Nerve growth factor and forskolin prevent H202-induced apoptosis in PC 12 cells by glutathione independent mechanism. Neuroscience Letters. 1996;**212**:179-182

[71] Ronemus M, Iossifov I, Levy D, Wigler M. The role of de novo mutations in the genetics of autism spectrum disorders. Nature Reviews. Genetics. 2014;2:133-141

[72] Mottron L, Belleville S, Guy A, Rouleau OC. Linking neocortical, cognitive, and genetic variability in autism with alterations of brain plasticity: The trigger-threshold-target model. Neuroscience and Biobehavioral Reviews. 2014;15:1-10

[73] Sharma SS. Emerging neuroprotective approaches in stroke treatment. Crips. 2003;4(4):8-12

From Neuronal Differentiation of iPSCs to 3D Neural Organoids: Modeling of Neurodegenerative Diseases

Matteo Bordoni, Valentina Fantini,
Orietta Pansarasa and Cristina Cereda

Additional information is available at the end of the chapter

http://dx.doi.org/10.5772/intechopen.80055

Abstract

In the last decade, the finding that somatic cells can be reprogrammed into induced pluripotent stem cells (iPSCs) leads to a great improvement of research involving the use of differentiated stem cells as model of diseases. In the field of neurodegeneration, iPSC technology allowed to culture in vitro all the types of patient-specific neurons, not only helping the discovery of diseases' etiopathology but also testing new drugs with a personalized medicine approach. Moreover, iPSCs can be combined with the 3D bioprinting technology, allowing physiological cell-to-cell interactions, given by a combination of several biomaterials, scaffolds, and cells. This technology combines bioplotter and biomaterials which can encapsulate several types of cells, e.g., iPSCs or differentiated neurons, to develop an innovative cellular model. iPSCs and 3D cell cultures' technologies represent the first step to obtain a more reliable model, like an organoid to facilitate neurodegenerative diseases' investigation.

Keywords: cell culture, iPSCs, 3D bioprinting, disease modeling, personalized medicine

1. Introduction

Stem cells represent an unlimited cell source because of their property of self-renewal, and they can also differentiate into almost all adult cell types thanks to their pluripotency characteristic [1]. One of the main problems of stem cell research was the invasively harvesting techniques, such as through bone marrow, adipose tissue extraction by liposuction, or blood apheresis [2]. In 2006, the discovery that adult somatic cells can be reprogrammed into the so-called induced pluripotent stem cells (iPSCs) has allowed to generate stem cell lines with minimally invasive techniques, like skin biopsy or, more recently, blood withdrawal [3]. These recent findings has led to an outstanding increase in disease mechanisms and drug screening studies involving stem cells, in particular for neurodegenerative diseases because of the impossibility to obtain neural cells from patients. The ability to reprogram patient-specific cells also opens new opportunities for the personalized medicine approach of drug discovery. Moreover, the development of 3D bioprinting provided a useful tool to generate innovative cell cultures, permitting to have a 3D model in which cells can be disposed with a controlled manner and where they can grow in a tissue-like structures [4]. Obviously, 3D bioprinting opened new possibilities in the field of tissue engineering, but it can be helpful also for disease modeling. In fact, the generation of a 3D scaffold that can resemble the human tissues will permit to study neurodegenerative diseases in the so-called brain in dish. Finally, the combination of 3D bioprinting technique with iPSC technology will permit to develop one of the most realistic and reliable in vitro cell cultures, permitting to study organoids with patients' differentiated cells, leading to a personalized medicine approach in drug testing.

2. Stem cells

Stem cell research is considered one of the most promising areas in cell biology and regenerative medicine due to stem cells' unique properties of self-renewing and differentiation into all types of cells. These cells represent nowadays the main tool in the regenerative medicine field because they permit to generate cells needed for transplantation in several degenerative diseases [1], such as rheumatoid arthritis [5], diabetes mellitus [6], heart failure [7], liver diseases [8], and neurological disorders [9–11]. Moreover, stem cells represent an important tool for modeling human diseases, in particular for diseases that affect cells that cannot be easily collected and cultivated. One of the biggest issues in the study of neurodegenerative diseases is the lack of good cellular models that recapitulate the mechanisms underlying their pathophysiology, and in the last decade, stem cells played a major role in the study of these diseases.

2.1. Embryonic stem cells

The first evidence that human stem cells, called human embryonic stem cells (hESC), could be derived from a 5-day blastocyst was reported in 1998 by Thomson and colleagues [12]. ES cells have the ability to proliferate indefinitely and are considered pluripotent cells because they can differentiate into all three germ layers (ectoderm, mesoderm, and endoderm) and, thus, they can generate all the differentiated cells of the adult [13, 14]. Despite that they helped stem cell research, they also opened many controversies because ES cells are obtained from blastocyst, killing the fertilized embryo that has the potential to generate a human being [15]. The big ethical issue on the use of hES cells encouraged researchers to understand the pathways underlying the staminality of this kind of cells.

2.2. Induced pluripotent stem cells

The research done with ES cells and the finding of their highly expressed transcription factors, permitted in 2006 to induce mouse's fibroblasts to become pluripotent, by retrovirus-mediated transduction with four transcription factors, i.e., Oct-3/4, Sox2, KLF4, and c-Myc [16]. The following studies allowed to improve the technique, permitting to generate induced pluripotent stem cells (iPSCs) from adult human cells and to reprogram cells from several tissues [15]. Moreover, it is now possible to generate iPS cells by different transduction methods (**Figure 1**), using different viral and nonviral constructs, as well as integrative and non-integrative system approaches [17]. The best methods to reprogram cells are the non-integrative methods, and the four main groups are available: non-integrative viral delivery, episomal delivery, RNA delivery, and protein delivery [18]. The establishment of human iPS cells has led to have an unlimited source of stem cells overcoming the ethical limit of hES cells. Moreover, iPSCs can be reprogrammed from any somatic cell line of the patients providing a way to study diseases' mechanisms potentially for each patient, opening to the so-called personalized medicine (**Figure 1**). Actually, many iPSCs' lines have been generated from patients with neurodegenerative disease, like Alzheimer's disease (AD) [19], Parkinson's disease (PD) [20], amyotrophic lateral sclerosis (ALS) [21], and Huntington's disease (HD) [22].

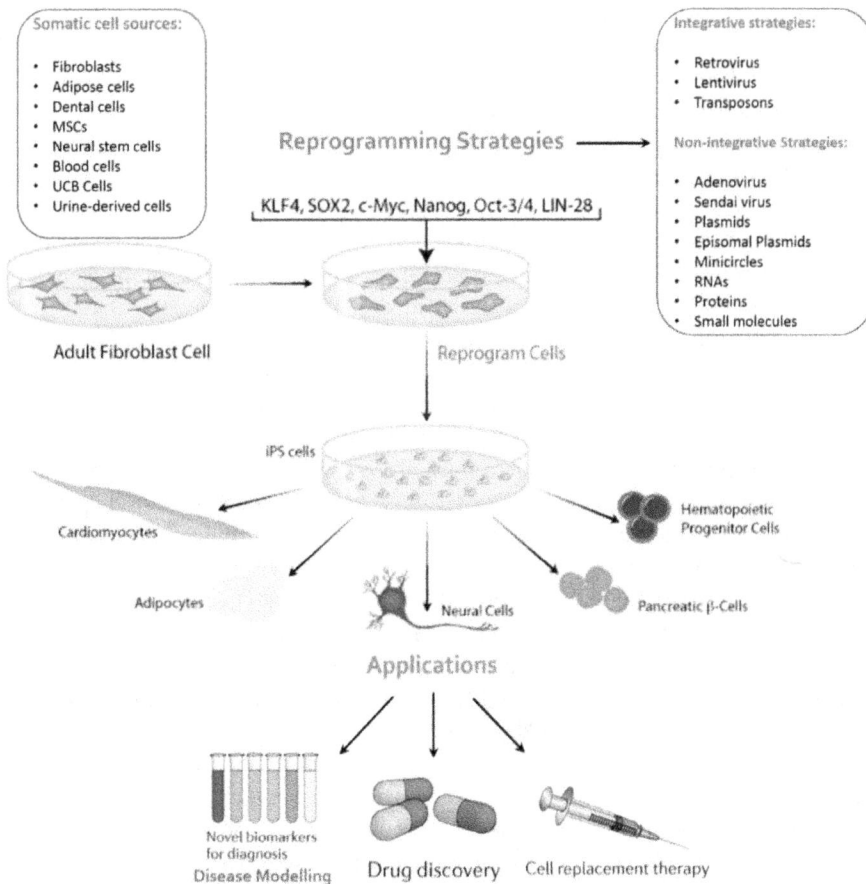

Figure 1. An overview of iPSC technology. Somatic cells can be taken from several sources, like the skin, blood, and urine. There are many reprogramming strategies, and the best ones are the non-integrative strategies. iPSCs can be differentiated into diverse cell lines that can be used for disease modeling, for drug discovery, and for cell replacement therapy (the image was taken from Sharma [23]).

2.2.1. iPSCs in Alzheimer's disease

Alzheimer's disease (AD) is the most common form of dementia and is characterized by the progressive loss of memory and cognitive functions. The disease leads to a severe form of dementia that causes the death of the patient [24]. The two main hallmarks of the disease are the accumulation of amyloid beta (Aβ) plaques in the extracellular compartment and the aggregation of the tau protein in the intracellular compartment. Only 1–5% of AD cases have a genetic cause, while in the other cases, the real pathogenesis is still unknown [25].

Many groups used and performed several studies on in vitro models with neural and nonneuronal cells derived from iPSCs. For example, higher susceptibility to Aβ1–Aβ42 oligomers was found in neuronal precursors derived from iPSC (iPSCs-NSCs) of a patient with a mutation in the PSEN1 gene (PSEN1-A246E mutation) compared to sporadic AD patient and healthy control [26]. The authors concluded that neurons derived from AD iPSCs could be effective in drug screening, to develop new treatments that protect cells from the toxicity of the Aβ peptides in the AD brain [26]. A similar result was obtained with iPSC-derived neurons of sporadic AD patients and of a patient carrying the pathogenic APP-E693Δ mutation. The study shows that these cell lines produce intracellular Aβ oligomers, resulting in a good cellular model of AD [27]. iPSCs can be used to find new potential biomarkers of the disease, as suggested by Shirotani et al. that developed an innovative method on neurons differentiated from iPSCs [28]. Moreover, induced fAD mutations by genome editing of neurons derived from healthy controls could resemble the pathophysiology of the disease. A decrease in endocytosis and soma-to-axon transcytosis of LDL was found in human neurons with expression of PSEN1ΔE9 induced with genome editing technology. To confirm the potential role of iPSCs in drug discovery, the authors reported that defects were rescued by β-secretase inhibition [29]. Another study reported the generation of an Alzheimer-related protein association network using iPSCs, demonstrating that they can be used as drug screening model and finding a reduction of tau protein after treatment with an inhibitor of γ-secretase [30]. For drug testing, it is important that iPSC-derived neurons are well differentiated, because it was seen that between early and late differentiation stages, cells have different susceptibilities to drugs [31]. Genome editing technology could be used also for mutations' correction, generating an isogenic control. For example, Pires and colleagues reported that A79V-iPSC line in combination of A79V-GC-iPSC line could be used to study pathological cellular phenotypes related to A79V mutation in PSEN [32]. Interestingly, the role of iPSCs in AD research was supported also by analyzing neurons derived from iPSCs of patients with Down syndrome that usually have a high risk of developing AD early. Authors found that such neural cells reproduce AD-like initial cellular hallmark, resulting useful for modeling this variant of AD [33]. Finally, also nonneuronal cells derived from iPSCs could be very useful in disease modeling and drug screening. Many pathological hallmarks were found aberrant in astrocytes derived from iPSCs of fAD and sAD patients suggesting that astrocytic atrophy could be a plausible mechanism for early cognitive impairment and thus opening new therapeutic strategies for AD intervention [34]. Another study reported changes in PSEN1-mutated iPSC-derived astrocytes, revealing the major role of such cells and confirming the importance to implement iPSC technology to support neurodegenerative diseases' study [35].

These researches suggest that iPSC-derived neurons from AD patients can help not only to unravel disease's mechanisms but also to screen new treatment and to find new possible drug targets. Moreover, the authors hypothesize that gene correction is a useful tool to generate isogenic controls or to induce AD mutations in healthy controls. Finally, iPSCs can be differentiated into glial cells, e.g., astrocytes, which in recent years gain an important role in the pathogenesis of several neurodegenerative diseases.

2.2.2. iPSCs in Parkinson's disease

Parkinson's disease (PD) is the second most common neurodegenerative disease after AD, with a prevalence of 1% out of the individuals over age 60 years and 4% of the population with an age over 85 years [36]. The most common mutations, found in about 10% of Parkinson's patients, are present in six genes: SNCA, LRRK2, Parkin, PINK1, DJ-1, and ATP13A2 [37].

Usually, iPSCs are differentiated into dopaminergic (DA) neurons to model PD because the disease is characterized by the loss of DA neurons of the *substantia nigra* in the midbrain. Since monogenic mutations cause an idiopathic-like disease, diverse iPSC lines of patients with Parkin and PINK1 mutations (e.g., 2–4 exon deletions of Parkin and PINK1 Q456X) have been developed. It was seen that these cell lines present abnormalities in mitochondrial and dopamine homoeostasis, microtubular stability, and axonal outgrowth, resulting in an optimal model of the disease [38]. For example, many PD cell phenotypes, i.e., mitochondrial dysfunction, elevated α-synuclein, synaptic dysfunction, DA accumulation, and increased oxidative stress and ROS, were found in iPSC-DA neurons of patients carrying mutations in parkin (V324A) and PINK1 (Q456X) genes [39]. The role in neurons' maturation of elevated α-synuclein caused by SNCA gene triplication was investigated in a cellular model obtained from PD-derived iPSCs. The author has claimed that such triplication leads to the impairment of differentiation and maturation of iPSCs [40]. An electrophysiological characterization of control dopaminergic neurons derived from iPSC was provided by Hartfield and colleagues that confirmed that these cells have the physiological hallmarks of dopaminergic neurons previously reported only on rodent slice. These results suggested that such cells can be considered a useful tool for the physiological study of PD [41]. Moreover, several evidences suggest that PD is not only a brain disease but also a gastrointestinal disorder; thus, Son and colleagues differentiated iPSCs carrying an LRRK2 G2019S mutation in both neural and intestinal phenotypes, providing the first evidence that G2019S mutation causes significant changes in gene expression also in the intestinal cells [42]. Interestingly, the pathologic phenotype was reversed in cortical neurons derived from iPSCs of patients mutated in SNCA using a small molecule found by yeast screening, opening new possibilities in drug screening and testing [43]. Finally, iPSCs have allowed an innovative co-culture of microglial cells and cortical neurons, displaying a unique cytokine profile impossible to obtain without iPSCs [44]. iPSCs were proposed to be used for tissue transplantation, and Kikuchi et al. achieved the transplantation of human iPS cell-derived dopaminergic neurons in a primate model of PD treated with MTPT. The authors reported an increase in spontaneous movement of the monkeys, demonstrating for the first time that such transplantation could be clinically applicable for the treatment of PD patients [45].

The studies previously reported hypothesize that iPSC-derived neurons from PD patients can be very useful in the research of PD pathophysiology and to find new therapeutic targets for innovative drugs. Moreover, the possibility to differentiate iPSCs into nonneuronal cells, such as microglial and intestinal cells, will help to unravel the role of immunity response and the gastrointestinal disorder that affect PD patients.

2.2.3. iPSCs in amyotrophic lateral sclerosis

Amyotrophic lateral sclerosis (ALS) is the most prevalent motor neuron disease and is characterized by the progressive loss of upper and lower motor neurons (MNs), leading to muscle atrophy, paralysis, and finally death usually after 2–5 years from the first diagnosis [21]. Also for ALS the cause is still unknown, but in about 5–10% of cases, several genes are found mutated, among which are SOD1, TARDPB, and FUS [46]. Moreover, in 2013 the GGGGCC-hexanucleotide repeat expansion in C9orf72 locus was found in many familial and sporadic cases of ALS [47].

MNs derived from iPSCs are the most common neural cell type used in ALS involving the use of stem cell differentiation. For example, an increase in oxidative stress and in DNA damage was found in iPSC-derived C9ORF72 MNs, confirming that the reduction of oxidative stress could help to delay patients' death [48]. Moreover, MNs derived from iPSCs with induced mutation in FUS (P525L) were used to investigate the transcriptome and microRNA, finding an alteration of both in pathways with implications for ALS pathogenesis [49]. The role of astrocytes was also investigated in both sporadic and VCP mutant patients, suggesting that in ALS patients, the co-culture between MNs and astrocytes causes alterations in both cell types [50, 51]. Moreover, the genetic correction allowed to study pathways implicated in ALS, like Bhinge and colleagues that found that the activation of AP1 drives neurodegeneration in genetic corrected SOD1 mutant MNs [52]. Small-molecule compounds that regulate IGF-2 expression were found to increase MN resilience, screening the compounds in iPSC-derived MNs [53]. Another example is given by Egawa and colleagues that firstly generated and characterized MNs from iPSCs of patients carrying TDP-43 mutations. They found some pathological hallmark, such as short neurites and abnormal-insoluble TDP-43. Then, they tested trichostatin A, spliceostatin A, garcinol, and anacardic acid and found that the last one, an inhibitor of histone deacetylase, rescued the pathogenic abnormalities like TDP-43 mRNA [54]. All these researches suggest the increasing importance of iPSCs as model for drug screening.

These works suggest that MNs derived from iPSCs of mutated and sporadic ALS patients can be a helpful tool to study both disease mechanisms and drug screening. Several investigations can be done in iPSC-derived MN cellular models, e.g., oxidative stress, DNA damage, and transcriptome. The co-culture between astrocytes and MNs can give information about how they interact with each other and whether this interaction could have a pathophysiologic role in ALS.

2.2.4. iPSCs in Huntington's disease

Huntington's disease (HD) is characterized by loss of neurons mainly in the caudate nucleus, the putamen, and the cerebral cortex with affection in a later stage of other areas, e.g., the hippocampus and hypothalamus [55]. Despite other neurodegenerative diseases, the cause of HD is well known; in fact it is an autosomal dominant genetic disorder caused by an expansion mutation of the trinucleotide (CAG) repeat in the HTT (IT15) gene, encoding a 350-kDa protein called Huntingtin (HTT) [56]. Even though the genetic cause is clear, the mechanisms through which mutant HTT results in the degeneration of some types of neurons are still unclear. Thus, studies on HD models are needed in order to discover treatments.

As the neurodegenerative diseases previously reported, also for HD, neurons differentiated from iPSCs of patients helped to understand the role of mutant HTT gene and the mechanisms that lead to the pathology. For example, early molecular changes in intracellular signaling, expression of oxidative stress proteins, and p53 pathway both in iPSCs and in neurons differentiated from them were reported [57]. Another study reported changes in neuronal development and adult neurogenesis, exploiting the iPSC capacity to model also embryonal development [58]. The generation of iPSCs from a patient that presents an expansion in the HTT gene without any symptom is very intriguing. The generation of iPSCs in an early stage of HD will allow to study the pathological process and the abnormal changes that lead to the pathology [59]. The possibility to differentiate iPSCs into neurons opened the possibility to discover new therapeutic targets, e.g., pre-mRNA trans-splicing modules [60]. Finally, the role of glial cells was investigated in several studies, among these who studied it were Hsiao and colleagues that reported that HD astrocytes provide less pericyte coverage by promoting angiogenesis and reducing the number of pericytes [61]. Finally, in a mouse cell model of HD, many but not all pathological hallmarks of HD were found. This result suggests that nonhuman iPSCs must be used carefully when translated into human pathology [62].

The researches previously reported highlight the importance to have a realistic model of the disease to study mechanisms that lead to neurodegeneration and iPSC-derived neurons that represent as a useful tool. They can be used also to perform a study of drug discovery and drug screening, to better understand the effect of chemicals in neurons. Moreover, the possibility to differentiate iPSCs in nonneuronal cells, such as astrocytes, helps to discover the role of glial cells in HD pathogenesis.

3. 3D bioprinting

The term bioprinting was used for the first time in 2009 by Mironov with the release of the first issue of the journal *Biofabrication*, a magazine that took its name from the eponymous term biofabrication. While the term biofabrication is intended to indicate natural processes such as biomineralization, the term bioprinting is defined by Guillemot in 2010 as [63, 64].

The use of computer-aided transfer processes for patterning and assembling living and non-living materials with a prescribed 2D or 3D organization in order to produce bio-engineered structures serving in regenerative medicine, pharmacokinetic and basic cell biology studies.

3D bioprinting is an emerging technology, used for the manufacture and the generation of artificial tissues and organs [65], adding new approaches to tissue engineering (TE) and regenerative medicine, such as the manufacture of scaffold to support cells, as well as in situ deposition of cell suspensions [63]. Bioprinting technology has allowed to overcome several limits, such as the control of in vitro 3D biological structures and cellular distribution [66].

Bioprinting, through the use of hardware and software, has been used in particular for the design of three-dimensional structures, allowing the creation of "organoids" for biological and pharmacological studies, and to repair and replace human tissues.

3.1. Bioprinting and bioplotter techniques

Bioprinting can be distinguished on the basis of the bioink printing technique, allowing to change the printing processes according to the needs that the different cell types require: ink-jet, laser, and extrusion (**Figure 2**) [65]. In addition to the specific printer characteristic, each bioplotter must have common functionalities. The most important is the presence of a robotic displacement system that can move along the three Cartesian axes, x, y, and, for the 3D characteristics, z. Usually, the bioink is extruded from a dispenser, but it is possible to have more dispensers, permitting to have different bioinks in the same scaffold. One of the most recent techniques allows a coaxial extrusion, with a bioink that is surrounded by a second bioink. The sterility of the printout is usually guaranteed by the presence of sterile chamber with laminar flow system. If the bioplotter is quite small, this problem could be overcome by simply placing the bioprinter under a classic cellular hood. Finally, the presence of a dedicated software for the supply of bioink and for the high-resolution control of the design of the construct to be printed is essential [65].

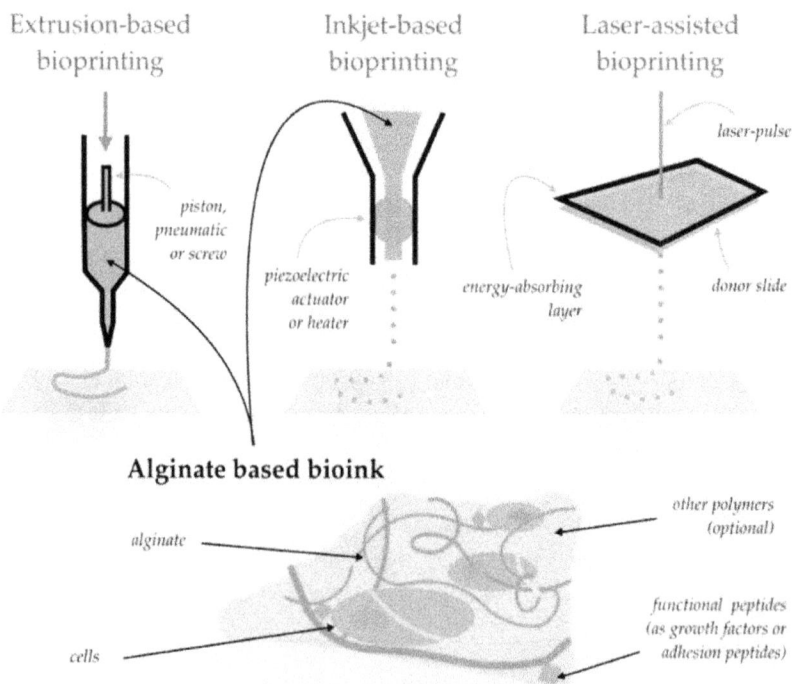

Figure 2. On the top the most used printing processes are extrusion-based (performed by piston, pneumatic method, or screw), inkjet-based operated by a piezoelectric actuator, and laser-assisted (composed of an energy-absorbing slide and a donor slide that collect the discharged bioink droplets). On the bottom the complexity of the 3D bioprinted construct, composed of a natural biocompatible material (e.G., alginate), cells, functional peptides, and other biocompatible materials. (the image was taken from Axpe and Oyen [67]).

First, bioplotters that appeared on the market were intended for a purely industrial use, since they had a high price. The costs limited their development and related researches. With the advent of technology and knowledge of bioprinting, we have witnessed the birth of multiple models of bioplotters, each with characteristics that reflect the needs of the individual creator [12, 13], e.g., increasing the number of nozzles for simultaneous extrusion of several materials [68] and changing the type of technology that controls the nozzle.

3.1.1. Inkjet bioplotter

Inkjet bioplotter was the first technique used in the 1980s in offices and then for domestic use. It was readapted around the year 2000 to be used as a biological printer, replacing the normal ink with a bioink, containing cells and biocompatible materials [69]. Droplets of the biomaterial are extruded from very small orifices, deposited on a substrate, maintaining good cell dispersion, viability, and functionality, even with different cellular types [70]. The stream can be continuous, command-driven (drop on demand), and electrodynamic. Both piezoelectric and thermal inkjet printers have been readapted for biological printing, offering many advantages in terms of simplicity, versatility, and material control, both in terms of quantity and speed in the printing process [71].

3.1.2. Laser technology

Laser-based direct writing was introduced in 1999 and is one of the most used laser-based bioprinting techniques [72]. The technique involves a layer with biological material (donor layer) and a layer that collect cells (acceptor layer) that are pushed by the laser through the first layer. The pulsation of the laser creates bubbles which in turn generate a shockwave, forcing the cells to pass from the donor layer to the acceptor layer. This technique allows to have a good resolution but has some disadvantages, such as irreversible damage to the cells because of the heat and light generated by the laser [65].

3.1.3. Extrusion-based bioprinter

The advent of TE has allowed extrusion technology to be thoroughly studied and applied to the field of bioprinting, for the generation of living tissues. Extrusion technique includes a combination of different delivery systems combined with an automatic robotic system for extrusion and 3D printing [73]. Deposition of the material takes place through extrusion to form a cylindrical filament made of a biocompatible gelatinous material, in which the cells are encapsulated, maintaining the desired three-dimensional structure [74]. This type of extrusion can be pneumatic or mechanical. Mechanical extrusion involves the use of a piston, which guides the deposit of the material allowing a good flow control through the nozzle, or a screw, which allows the extrusion of more viscous substances, but which can cause leakage of pressure, causing damage to cells. This technique also has some limits, particularly during the development of the biomaterial which must have the right viscosity to be extruded and the ability to be easily homogenized with cell suspension and to maintain three-dimensional structure [65].

3.2. Hydrogel and bioink

One of the fundamental elements that characterize the bioprinting process is the development of biomaterial, which must have specific characteristics: biocompatibility, printability, and ability to maintain a three-dimensional structure once printed and maintained in culture [65]. The main feature of the hydrogel, biocompatible material used as a three-dimensional support for cell growth, is the ability to be extremely hydrophilic, making it an excellent candidate in terms of biocompatibility for its use in bioprinting. It was initially used in TE because it was able to simulate the extracellular matrix, guarantying cell growth and communication [75]. Biomaterials are divided, According to their derivation, biomaterials are divided in natural or synthetic compunds. There are naturally derived polymers such as sodium alginate, gelatin, collagen, chitosan, fibrin, and GelMA [76–78] and synthetic polymers such as Pluronic®, polyethylene glycol (PEG), and polyurethanes [79, 80]. Over time, it has been seen how the natural compounds are more performing when placed in contact with the cells than the synthetic ones. Several cell types associated with different biomaterials to compose the bioink have already been used in several research areas, where cellular viability and motility have been demonstrated, as well as a spatial organization similar to in vivo tissue [81]. To create a new biomaterial, we must consider different physical, mechanical, and biological characteristics that are close to the tissue we want to recreate. Thus, researchers tend to create a combination of biomaterials for each cell type, and with well-defined printability specifications, so as to make the process as standardized and reproducible as possible, despite being a very open field and full of new developments. New-generation bioinks are now able to maintain each of these characteristics, thus improving the success in terms of bioprinting. All this is possible if particular attention is paid to the following chemical, physical, and biological properties: rheological studies (viscosity, thinning, viscoelasticity), biofunctional analysis, biodegradation, and polymerization (cytocompatibility, cell adhesion, migration, proliferation, and differentiation) [82]. One of the most important features that has different biomaterials is the ability to cross-link once the bioink has been printed, reticulating the bioink in which cells are encapsulated, without affecting the viability, the differentiation, and the capacity of migration [83]. The ability to polymerize depends on the material used; for example, collagen needs chemical cross-link, through covalent bonds that bind free amines or carboxylic groups of collagen that is able to reticulate, also through a biological process, and through the interaction with transglutaminase. Other compounds, such as sodium alginate, use an ionic cross-link: divalent cations such as Ca^{2+} bind to two sodium alginate residues, cross-linking the structure. UV radiation is a very promising cross-link technique given its reaction speed but with many questions regarding the possible damage induced to the cells included in the material. Other materials, such as gelatin and agarose, are heat-sensitive, so they are used during the printing process at the melting temperature and then stiffened with cooling [84–87]. One of the most common types of bioink used in bioprinting techniques is the so-called cell-laden hydrogel, which includes natural hydrogels such as agarose, sodium alginate, chitosan, collagen, gelatin, fibrin, and hyaluronic acid and synthetic hydrogels such as Pluronic® and PEG. Hydrogels can be used with the most common bioplotter that mount different printing techniques, allowing the creation of bioinks that combine the advantages of the natural material with the advantages of synthetic materials [88]. Recent findings have shown also the possibility to transfect cells with target DNA or plasmid, directly during the bioprinting process [80]. A new promising method to develop bioinks is the base on decellularized extracellular matrix. This kind of bioink consists in eliminating cells from a tissue of interest, keeping intact the extracellular matrix that is then pulverized and subsequently used as bioink once dissolved in a saline buffer. Finally, the cell suspension bioinks, characterized by a print that does not have a support material, like a scaffold, are also very common. It uses aggregates of cells in culture medium, placed in mono- or multicell spheres [73]. This technique is based on the liquidity of the tissue and its fusion, such as to allow cells to assemble, merge, and create cell-to-cell interconnections [89, 90]. Organovo was the first medical research company that used this technique to create functional human tissues. They developed a liver model using parenchyma cells and an extrusion printer of their own creation [91].

4. 3D bioprinting and neurodegeneration

In the last decade, the possibility of replacing dead cells in degenerative processes affecting the central nervous system opened the way for a more intense and accurate study of stem cells and their possibility of replacing damaged tissue [92]. It was also thought to exploit the ability of stem cells to secrete cytokines and growth factors, offering benefits such as anti-inflammatory effects, protection of neural cells, and endogenous recovery systems. Transplanting these cells into damaged sites presents various problems such as low cell survival and limited engraftment [93]. To minimize these problems, it was decided to use three-dimensional scaffold printing that mimics the complexity both from the biological and functional points of view of the tissue to be replaced [94].

The manufacture of three-dimensional prefabricated scaffolds has already given positive results in the treatment and repair of spinal and nerve damage but with a great limitation in terms of control of the external shape of the scaffold and of its internal architecture [95, 96]. These problems have been overcome with the 3D bioprinting, which leaves the operator complete freedom regarding the shape, the material, and its internal architecture. The recent developments in the field of 3D bioprinting are mostly aimed to the field of regenerative medicine, to respond to the growing demand for tissues and organs for transplants, arriving only later for this technology to be applied to basic scientific research. Until now only few studies have focused on using 3D printing applied to the creation of neural tissue compared to other widely studied tissues such as the skin, bones, heart tissue, and cartilaginous structures [97]. The few studies published so far, in which they use nerve cells in 3D printing processes [98, 99], show a poor characterization of bioinks to be used for nerve cells, due to the delicacy of the tissue to be recreated and of the characteristics necessary for the optimal growth of the nervous tissue [94]. Recently, researchers also think that the nervous tissue printed in 3D may be used for the neural regeneration, a huge possibility in the field of neurodegeneration to replace degenerated neural tissue [78, 80].

The creation of nerve tissue by bioprinting is also used for pharmacological studies, for toxicological screening, and for basic research. It is necessary to underline how this field is still in its infancy and how it is necessary to validate this model for the applications described up to now, to be sure that the model completely recapitulates the pathophysiology that we want to investigate with this tool [94] in particular with regard to neurodegenerative diseases.

5. Conclusions

In the last decade, two groundbreaking discoveries, i.e., somatic cell reprogramming into iPSCs and 3D bioprinting, changed the way to modeling diseases, in particular for those pathologies which are hard to study in simple cell cultures, such as neurodegenerative diseases. The first one is permitted to obtain neural cell cultures in few months starting from adult somatic cells, like fibroblasts and PBMCs, while 3D bioprinting consists in the print of hydrogel and cells, to generate models that imitate tissue characteristics. While iPSCs are differentiated into neurons in many papers for disease modeling, 3D bioprinting is actually used for few tissues, like the cartilage, bone, and heart. Neural 3D cell cultures are still in development, there are no target bioinks, and the studies that combine neuronal cells and 3D bioprinting are more complicated than other tissues because of the fragility of such cells. Despite this hurdle, the possibility to create an in vitro neural tissue would open many fields of research that today are unreachable, first of all the opportunity to study the 3D spatial connection between different neuronal populations and how they communicate with each other. In combination with iPSC technology, we can create a physiological model to understand physiological and pathological mechanisms and to better understand mechanisms underlying neurodegenerative diseases.

Finally, the combination between 3D bioprinting and iPSC technology will open not only new possibilities in many fields, drug screening, replacing expensive in vivo experiments, and overcoming animal models' issues, but also personalized medicine thanks to the use of cells derived from patients. More intriguingly, the generation of a 3D neural tissue composed of patient's cell will allow the so-called neuro-regeneration, opening the possibility to replace a degenerated tissue.

Conflict of interest

The authors declare that there is no conflict of interest.

Author details

Matteo Bordoni[1,2], Valentina Fantini[1], Orietta Pansarasa[1] and Cristina Cereda[1*]

*Address all correspondence to: cristina.cereda@mondino.it

1 Genomic and post-Genomic Center, Mondino Foundation, Pavia, Italy

2 Department of Brain and Behavioural Sciences, University of Pavia, Pavia, Italy

References

[1] Lodi D, Iannitti T, Palmieri B. Stem cells in clinical practice: Applications and warnings. Journal of Experimental & Clinical Cancer Research. 2011;**30**:9

[2] Ong CS, Yesantharao P, Huang CY, Mattson G, Boktor J, Fukunishi T, Zhang H, Hibino N. 3D bioprinting using stem cells. Pediatric Research. 2017;**83**(1-2):223-231

[3] Haase A, Göhring G, Martin U. Generation of non-transgenic iPS cells from human cord blood CD34+ cells under animal component-free conditions. Stem Cell Research. 2017;**21**: 71-73

[4] Moroni L, Boland T, Burdick JA, De Maria C, Derby B, Forgacs G, Groll J, Li Q, Malda J, Mironov VA, et al. Biofabrication: A guide to technology and terminology. Trends in Biotechnology. 2017;**36**(4):384-402

[5] De Kleer IM, Brinkman DM, Ferster A, Abinun M, Quartier P, Van Der Net J, Ten Cate R, Wedderburn LR, et al. Autologous stem cell transplantation for refractory juvenile idiopathic arthritis: Analysis of clinical effects, mortality, and transplant related morbidity. Annals of the Rheumatic Diseases. 2004;**63**(10):1318-1326

[6] Trivedi HL, Vanikar AV, Thakker U, Firoze A, Dave SD, Patel CN, Patel JV, Bhargava AB, Shankar V. Human adipose tissue-derived mesenchymal stem cells combined with hematopoietic stem cell transplantation synthesize insulin. Transplantation Proceedings. 2008;**40**(4):1135-1139

[7] Schächinger V, Assmus B, Erbs S, Elsässer A, Haberbosch W, Hambrecht R, Yu J, Corti R, Mathey DG, Hamm CW, Tonn T, Dimmeler S, Zeiher AM, R.-A. investigators. Intracoronary infusion of bone marrow-derived mononuclear cells abrogates adverse left ventricular remodelling post-acute myocardial infarction: Insights from the reinfusion of enriched progenitor cells and infarct remodelling in acute myocardial infarction (REPAIR-AMI) trial. European Journal of Heart Failure. 2009;**11**(10):973-979

[8] Pai M, Zacharoulis D, Milicevic MN, Helmy S, Jiao LR, Levicar N, Tait P, Scott M, Marley SB, Jestice K, et al. Autologous infusion of expanded mobilized adult bone marrow-derived CD34+ cells into patients with alcoholic liver cirrhosis. The American Journal of Gastroenterology. 2008;**103**(8):1952-1958

[9] Papadeas ST, Maragakis NJ. Advances in stem cell research for amyotrophic lateral sclerosis. Current Opinion in Biotechnology. 2009;**20**(5):545-551

[10] Olanow CW, Gracies JM, Goetz CG, Stoessl AJ, Freeman T, Kordower JH, Godbold J, Obeso JA. Clinical pattern and risk factors for dyskinesias following fetal nigral transplantation in Parkinson's disease: A double blind video-based analysis. Movement Disorders. 2009;**24**(3):336-343

[11] Rosser AE, Barker RA, Harrower T, Watts C, Farrington M, Ho AK, Burnstein RM, Menon DK, Gillard JH, Pickard J, Dunnett SB. NEST-UK, unilateral transplantation of human primary fetal tissue in four patients with Huntington's disease: NEST-UK safety report ISRCTN no 36485475. Journal of Neurology, Neurosurgery, and Psychiatry. 2002;**73**(6): 678-685

[12] Thomson JA, Itskovitz-Eldor J, Shapiro SS, Waknitz MA, Swiergiel JJ, Marshall VS, Jones JM. Embryonic stem cell lines derived from human blastocysts. Science. 1998;**282**(5391):1145-1147

[13] Evans MJ, Kaufman MH. Establishment in culture of pluripotential cells from mouse embryos. Nature. 1981;**292**(5819):154-156

[14] Martin GR. Isolation of a pluripotent cell line from early mouse embryos cultured in medium conditioned by teratocarcinoma stem cells. Proceedings of the National Academy of Sciences of the United States of America. 1981;**78**(12):7634-7638

[15] Watt FM, Driskell RR. The therapeutic potential of stem cells. Philosophical Transactions of the Royal Society of London. Series B, Biological Sciences. 2010;**365**(1537):155-163

[16] Takahashi K, Yamanaka S. Induction of pluripotent stem cells from mouse embryonic and adult fibroblast cultures by defined factors. Cell. 2006;**126**(4):663-676

[17] Bahmad H, Hadadeh O, Chamaa F, Cheaito K, Darwish B, Makkawi AK, Abou-Kheir W. Modeling human neurological and neurodegenerative diseases: From induced pluripotent stem cells to neuronal differentiation and its applications in neurotrauma. Frontiers in Molecular Neuroscience. 2017;**10**:50

[18] González F, Boué S, Izpisúa Belmonte JC. Methods for making induced pluripotent stem cells: Reprogramming à la carte. Nature Reviews. Genetics. 2011;**12**(4):231-242

[19] Robbins JP, Price J. Human induced pluripotent stem cells as a research tool in Alzheimer's disease. Psychological Medicine. 2017;**47**(15):2587-2592

[20] Cobb MM, Ravisankar A, Skibinski G, Finkbeiner S. iPS cells in the study of PD molecular pathogenesis. Cell and Tissue Research. 2017;**373**(1):61-77

[21] Csobonyeiova M, Polak S, Nicodemou A, Danisovic L. Induced pluripotent stem cells in modeling and cell-based therapy of amyotrophic lateral sclerosis. Journal of Physiology and Pharmacology. 2017;**68**(5):649-657

[22] Tousley A, Kegel-Gleason KB. Induced pluripotent stem cells in Huntington's disease research: Progress and opportunity. Journal of Huntington's Disease. 2016;**5**(2):99-131

[23] Sharma R. iPS cells-the triumphs and tribulations. Dentistry Journal (Basel). 2016;**4**(2):19-42

[24] Karch CM, Cruchaga C, Goate AM. Alzheimer's disease genetics: From the bench to the clinic. Neuron. 2014;**83**(1):11-26

[25] Karch CM, Goate AM. Alzheimer's disease risk genes and mechanisms of disease pathogenesis. Biological Psychiatry. 2015;**77**(1):43-51

[26] Armijo E, Gonzalez C, Shahnawaz M, Flores A, Davis B, Soto C. Increased susceptibility to Aβ toxicity in neuronal cultures derived from familial Alzheimer's disease (PSEN1-A246E) induced pluripotent stem cells. Neuroscience Letters. 2017;**639**:74-81

[27] Kondo T, Asai M, Tsukita K, Kutoku Y, Ohsawa Y, Sunada Y, Imamura K, Egawa N, Yahata N, et al. Modeling Alzheimer's disease with iPSCs reveals stress phenotypes associated with intracellular Aβ and differential drug responsiveness. Cell Stem Cell. 2013;**12**(4):487-496

[28] Shirotani K, Matsuo K, Ohtsuki S, Masuda T, Asai M, Kutoku Y, Ohsawa Y, Sunada Y, Kondo T, Inoue H, Iwata N. A simplified and sensitive method to identify Alzheimer's disease biomarker candidates using patient-derived induced pluripotent stem cells (iPSCs). Journal of Biochemistry. 2017;**162**(6):391-394

[29] Woodruff G, Reyna SM, Dunlap M, Van Der Kant R, Callender JA, Young JE, Roberts EA, Goldstein LS. Defective transcytosis of APP and lipoproteins in human iPSC-derived neurons with familial Alzheimer's disease mutations. Cell Reports. 2016;17(3):759-773

[30] Hossini AM, Megges M, Prigione A, Lichtner B, Toliat MR, Wruck W, Schröter F, Nuernberg P, et al. Induced pluripotent stem cell-derived neuronal cells from a sporadic Alzheimer's disease donor as a model for investigating AD-associated gene regulatory networks. BMC Genomics. 2015;16:84

[31] Yahata N, Asai M, Kitaoka S, Takahashi K, Asaka I, Hioki H, Kaneko T, Maruyama K, Saido TC, Nakahata T, Asada T, Yamanaka S, Iwata N, Inoue H. Anti-Aβ drug screening platform using human iPS cell-derived neurons for the treatment of Alzheimer's disease. PLoS One. 2011;6(9):e25788

[32] Pires C, Schmid B, Petræus C, Poon A, Nimsanor N, Nielsen TT, Waldemar G, Hjermind LE, Nielsen JE, Hyttel P, Freude KK. Generation of a gene-corrected isogenic control cell line from an Alzheimer's disease patient iPSC line carrying a A79V mutation in PSEN1. Stem Cell Research. 2016;17(2):285-288

[33] Dashinimaev EB, Artyuhov AS, Bolshakov AP, Vorotelyak EA, Vasiliev AV. Neurons derived from induced pluripotent stem cells of patients with down syndrome reproduce early stages of Alzheimer's disease type pathology in vitro. Journal of Alzheimer's Disease. 2017;56(2):835-847

[34] Jones VC, Atkinson-Dell R, Verkhratsky A, Mohamet L. Aberrant iPSC-derived human astrocytes in Alzheimer's disease. Cell Death & Disease. 2017;8(3):e2696

[35] Oksanen M, Petersen AJ, Naumenko N, Puttonen K, Lehtonen Š, Gubert Olivé M, Shakirzyanova A, et al. PSEN1 mutant iPSC-derived model reveals severe astrocyte pathology in Alzheimer's disease. Stem Cell Reports. 2017;9(6):1885-1897

[36] Domingo A, Klein C. Genetics of Parkinson disease. Handbook of Clinical Neurology. 2018;147:211-227

[37] Klein C, Westenberger A. Genetics of Parkinson's disease. Cold Spring Harbor Perspectives in Medicine. 2012;2(1):a008888

[38] Rakovic A, Seibler P, Klein C. iPS models of Parkin and PINK1. Biochemical Society Transactions. 2015;43(2):302-307

[39] Chung SY, Kishinevsky S, Mazzulli JR, Graziotto J, Mrejeru A, Mosharov EV, Puspita L, Valiulahi P, et al. Parkin and PINK1 patient iPSC-derived midbrain dopamine neurons exhibit mitochondrial dysfunction and α-Synuclein accumulation. Stem Cell Reports. 2016;7(4):664-677

[40] Oliveira LM, Falomir-Lockhart LJ, Botelho MG, Lin KH, Wales P, Koch JC, Gerhardt E, Taschenberger H, et al. Elevated α-synuclein caused by SNCA gene triplication impairs neuronal differentiation and maturation in Parkinson's patient-derived induced pluripotent stem cells. Cell Death & Disease. 2015;6:e1994

[41] Hartfield EM, Yamasaki-Mann M, Ribeiro Fernandes HJ, Vowles J, James WS, Cowley SA, Wade-Martins R. Physiological characterisation of human iPS-derived dopaminergic neurons. PLoS One. 2014;**9**(2):e87388

[42] Son MY, Sim H, Son YS, Jung KB, Lee MO, Oh JH, Chung SK, Jung CR, Kim J. Distinctive genomic signature of neural and intestinal organoids from familial Parkinson's disease patient-derived induced pluripotent stem cells. Neuropathology and Applied Neurobiology. 2017;**43**(7):584-603

[43] Chung CY, Khurana V, Auluck PK, Tardiff DF, Mazzulli JR, Soldner F, Baru V, Lou Y, Freyzon Y, et al. Identification and rescue of α-synuclein toxicity in Parkinson patient-derived neurons. Science. 2013;**342**(6161):983-987

[44] Haenseler W, Sansom SN, Buchrieser J, Newey SE, Moore CS, Nicholls FJ, Chintawar S, Schnell C, et al. A highly efficient human pluripotent stem cell microglia model displays a neuronal-co-culture-specific expression profile and inflammatory response. Stem Cell Reports. 2017;**8**(6):1727-1742

[45] Kikuchi T, Morizane A, Doi D, Magotani H, Onoe H, Hayashi T, Mizuma H, Takara S, Takahashi R, et al. Human iPS cell-derived dopaminergic neurons function in a primate Parkinson's disease model. Nature. 2017;**548**(7669):592-596

[46] Ludolph AC. Motor neuron disease: Genetic testing in amyotrophic lateral sclerosis. Nature Reviews. Neurology. 2017;**13**(5):262-263

[47] Mori K, Weng SM, Arzberger T, May S, Rentzsch K, Kremmer E, Schmid B, Kretzschmar HA, Cruts M, Van Broeckhoven C, Haass C, Edbauer D. The C9orf72 GGGGCC repeat is translated into aggregating dipeptide-repeat proteins in FTLD/ALS. Science. 2013;**339**(6125):1335-1338

[48] Lopez-Gonzalez R, Lu Y, Gendron TF, Karydas A, Tran H, Yang D, Petrucelli L, Miller BL, Almeida S, Gao FB. Poly(GR) in C9ORF72-related ALS/FTD compromises mitochondrial function and increases oxidative stress and DNA damage in iPSC-derived motor neurons. Neuron. 2016;**92**(2):383-391

[49] De Santis R, Santini L, Colantoni A, Peruzzi G, de Turris V, Alfano V, Bozzoni I, Rosa A. FUS mutant human motoneurons display altered transcriptome and microRNA pathways with implications for ALS pathogenesis. Stem Cell Reports. 2017;**9**(5):1450-1462

[50] Qian K, Huang H, Peterson A, Hu B, Maragakis NJ, Ming GL, Chen H, Zhang SC. Sporadic ALS astrocytes induce neuronal degeneration in vivo. Stem Cell Reports. 2017;**8**(4):843-855

[51] Hall CE, Yao Z, Choi M, Tyzack GE, Serio A, Luisier R, Harley J, Preza E, Arber C, Crisp SJ, Watson PMD, et al. Progressive motor neuron pathology and the role of astrocytes in a human stem cell model of VCP-related ALS. Cell Reports. 2017;**19**(9):1739-1749

[52] Bhinge A, Namboori SC, Zhang X, VanDongen AMJ, Stanton LW. Genetic correction of SOD1 mutant iPSCs reveals ERK and JNK activated AP1 as a driver of neurodegeneration in amyotrophic lateral sclerosis. Stem Cell Reports. 2017;**8**(4):856-869

[53] Osborn TM, Beagan J, Isacson O. Increased motor neuron resilience by small molecule compounds that regulate IGF-II expression. Neurobiology of Disease. 2018;**110**:218-230

[54] Egawa N, Kitaoka S, Tsukita K, Naitoh M, Takahashi K, Yamamoto T, Adachi F, Kondo T, et al. Drug screening for ALS using patient-specific induced pluripotent stem cells. Science Translational Medicine. 2012;**4**(145):145ra104

[55] Connor B. Concise review: The use of stem cells for understanding and treating Huntington's disease. Stem Cells. 2018;**36**(2):146-160

[56] A novel gene containing a trinucleotide repeat that is expanded and unstable on Huntington's disease chromosomes. The Huntington's disease collaborative research group. Cell. 1993;**72**(6):971-983

[57] Szlachcic WJ, Switonski PM, Krzyzosiak WJ, Figlerowicz M, Figiel M. Huntington disease iPSCs show early molecular changes in intracellular signaling, the expression of oxidative stress proteins and the p53 pathway. Disease Models & Mechanisms. 2015;**8**(9): 1047-1057

[58] H.i. Consortium. Developmental alterations in Huntington's disease neural cells and pharmacological rescue in cells and mice. Nature Neuroscience. 2017;**20**(5):648-660

[59] Bidollari E, Rotundo G, Ferrari D, Candido O, Bernardini L, Consoli F, De Luca A, Santimone I, Lamorte G, Ilari A, Squitieri F, Vescovi AL, Rosati J. Generation of induced pluripotent stem cell line, CSSi004-A (2962), from a patient diagnosed with Huntington's disease at the presymptomatic stage. Stem Cell Research. 2018;**28**:145-148

[60] Rindt H, Tom CM, Lorson CL, Mattis VB. Optimization of trans-splicing for Huntington's disease RNA therapy. Frontiers in Neuroscience. 2017;**11**:544

[61] Hsiao HY, Chen YC, Huang CH, Chen CC, Hsu YH, Chen HM, Chiu FL, Kuo HC, Chang C, Chern Y. Aberrant astrocytes impair vascular reactivity in Huntington disease. Annals of Neurology. 2015;**78**(2):178-192

[62] Castiglioni V, Onorati M, Rochon C, Cattaneo E. Induced pluripotent stem cell lines from Huntington's disease mice undergo neuronal differentiation while showing alterations in the lysosomal pathway. Neurobiology of Disease. 2012;**46**(1):30-40

[63] Guillemot F, Mironov V, Nakamura M. Bioprinting is coming of age: Report from the international conference on bioprinting and biofabrication in Bordeaux (3B'09). Biofabrication. 2010;**2**(1):010201

[64] Groll J, Boland T, Blunk T, Burdick JA, Cho D-W, Dalton PD, Derby B, Forgacs G, Li Q, Mironov VA, et al. Biofabrication: Reappraising the definition of an evolving field. Biofabrication. 2016;**8**(1):013001

[65] Dababneh AB, Ozbolat IT. Bioprinting technology: A current state-of-the-art review. Journal of Manufacturing Science and Engineering. 2014;**136**(6):061016

[66] Nakamura M, Iwanaga S, Henmi C, Arai K, Nishiyama Y. Biomatrices and biomaterials for future developments of bioprinting and biofabrication. Biofabrication. 2010; **2**(1):014110

[67] Axpe E, Oyen ML. Applications of alginate-based bioinks in 3D bioprinting. International Journal of Molecular Sciences. 2016;**17**(12):1976-1987

[68] Shim J-H, Lee J-S, Kim JY, Cho D-W. Bioprinting of a mechanically enhanced three-dimensional dual cell-laden construct for osteochondral tissue engineering using a multi-head tissue/organ building system. Journal of Micromechanics and Microengineering. 2012;**22**(8):085014-085014

[69] Wilson WC, Boland T. Cell and organ printing 1: Protein and cell printers. The Anatomical Record. 2003;**272A**(2):491-496

[70] Xu T, Jin J, Gregory C, Hickman JJ, Boland T. Inkjet printing of viable mammalian cells. Biomaterials. 2005;**26**(1):93-99

[71] Gudapati H, Dey M, Ozbolat I. A comprehensive review on droplet-based bioprinting: Past, present and future. Biomaterials. 2016;**102**:20-42

[72] Wang W, Li G, Huang Y. Modeling of bubble expansion-induced cell mechanical profile in laser-assisted cell direct writing. Journal of Manufacturing Science and Engineering. 2009;**131**(October):051013

[73] Mironov V. Printing technology to produce living tissue. Expert Opinion on Biological Therapy. 2003;**3**(5):701-704

[74] Ozbolat IT, Yu Y. Bioprinting toward organ fabrication: Challenges and future trends IEEE Transactions on Biomedical Engineering. 2015;**60**(November):691-699

[75] Patterson J, Martino MM, Hubbell JA. Biomimetic materials in tissue engineering. Materials Today. 2010;**13**(1-2):14-22

[76] Hunt NC, Grover LM. Cell encapsulation using biopolymer gels for regenerative medicine. Biotechnology Letters. 2010;**32**(6):733-742

[77] Brunger JM, Huynh NPT, Guenther CM, Perez-Pinera P, Moutos FT, Sanchez-Adams J, Gersbach CA, Guilak F. Scaffold-mediated lentiviral transduction for functional tissue engineering of cartilage. Proceedings of the National Academy of Sciences. 2014; **111**(9):E798-E806

[78] Zhou X, Cui H, Nowicki M, Miao S, Lee SJ, Masood F, Harris BT, Zhang LG. Three-dimensional-bioprinted dopamine-based matrix for promoting neural regeneration. ACS Applied Materials & Interfaces. 2018;**10**(10):8993-9001

[79] Censi R, Schuurman W, Malda J, Di Dato G, Burgisser PE, Dhert WJA, Van Nostrum CF, Di Martino P, Vermonden T, Hennink WE. A printable photopolymerizable thermosensitive p(HPMAm-lactate)-PEG hydrogel for tissue engineering. Advanced Functional Materials. 2011;**21**(10):1833-1842

[80] Ho L, Hsu SH. Cell reprogramming by 3D bioprinting of human fibroblasts in polyurethane hydrogel for fabrication of neural-like constructs. Acta Biomaterialia. 2018;**70**:57-70

[81] Lutolf MP, Gilbert PM, Blau HM. Designing materials to direct stem-cell fate. Nature. 2009;**462**(7272):433-441

[82] Kyle S, Jessop ZM, Al-Sabah A, Whitaker IS. Printability' of candidate biomaterials for extrusion based 3D printing: State-of-the-art. Advanced Healthcare Materials. 2017;**6**(16): 1-16

[83] Schütz K, Placht AM, Paul B, Brüggemeier S, Gelinsky M, Lode A. Three-dimensional plotting of a cell-laden alginate/methylcellulose blend: Towards biofabrication of tissue engineering constructs with clinically relevant dimensions. Journal of Tissue Engineering and Regenerative Medicine. 2017;**11**(5):1574-1587

[84] Cha C, Soman P, Zhu W, Nikkhah M, Camci-Unal G, Chen S, Khademhosseini A. Structural reinforcement of cell-laden hydrogels with microfabricated three dimensional scaffolds. Biomaterials Science. 2014;**2**(5):703-709

[85] Pereira RF, Bartolo PJ. Manufacturing of advanced biodegradable polymeric components. Journal of Applied Polymer Science. 2015;**132**(48)

[86] Rutz AL, Hyland KE, Jakus AE, Burghardt WR, Shah RN. A multi-material bioink method for 3D printing Tunable, Cel-compatible hydrogels. Advanced Materials. 2015;**27**(9): 1607-1614

[87] Skardal A, Devarasetty M, Kang HW, Mead I, Bishop C, Shupe T, Lee SJ, Jackson J, Yoo J, Soker S, Atala A. A hydrogel bioink toolkit for mimicking native tissue biochemical and mechanical properties in bioprinted tissue constructs. Acta Biomaterialia. 2015;**25**:24-34

[88] Ribeiro M, De Moraes MA, Beppu MM, Garcia MP, Fernandes MH, Monteiro FJ, Ferraz MP. Development of silk fibroin/nanohydroxyapatite composite hydrogels for bone tissue engineering. European Polymer Journal. 2015;**67**:66-77

[89] Jakab K, Neagu A, Mironov V, Markwald RR, Forgacs G. Engineering biological structures of prescribed shape using self-assembling multicellular systems. Proceedings of the National Academy of Sciences. 2004;**101**(9):2864-2869

[90] Fleming PA, Argraves WS, Gentile C, Neagu A, Forgacs G, Drake CJ. Fusion of uni-luminal vascular spheroids: A model for assembly of blood vessels. Developmental Dynamics. 2010;**239**(2):398-406

[91] Nguyen DG, Funk J, Robbins JB, Crogan-Grundy C, Presnell SC, Singer T, Roth AB. Bioprinted 3D primary liver tissues allow assessment of organ-level response to clinical drug induced toxicity in vitro. PLoS One. 2016;**11**(7):1-17

[92] Yoo J, Kim H-S, Hwang D-Y. Stem cells as promising therapeutic options for neurological disorders. Journal of Cellular Biochemistry. 2013;**114**(4):743-753

[93] Wu KH, Mo XM, Han ZC, Zhou B. Stem cell engraftment and survival in the ischemic heart. The Annals of Thoracic Surgery. 2011;**92**(5):1917-1925

[94] Hsieh F-Y, Hsu S-h. 3D bioprinting: A new insight into the therapeutic strategy of neural tissue regeneration. Organogenesis. 2015;**11**(4):153-158

[95] Panseri S, Cunha C, Lowery J, Del Carro U, Taraballi F, Amadio S, Vescovi A, Gelain F. Electrospun micro- and nanofiber tubes for functional nervous regeneration in sciatic nerve transections. BMC Biotechnology. 2008;**8**(1):39

[96] Cao H, Liu T, Chew SY. The application of nanofibrous scaffolds in neural tissue engineering. Advanced Drug Delivery Reviews. 2009;**61**(12):1055-1064

[97] Lee W, Pinckney J, Lee V, Lee J-H, Fischer K, Polio S, Park J-K, Yoo S-S. Three-dimensional bioprinting of rat embryonic neural cells. Neuroreport. 2009;**20**(8):798-803

[98] Lee YB, Polio S, Lee W, Dai G, Menon L, Carroll RS, Yoo SS. Bio-printing of collagen and VEGF-releasing fibrin gel scaffolds for neural stem cell culture. Experimental Neurology. 2010;**223**(2):645-652

[99] Lorber B, Hsiao W-K, Hutchings IM, Martin KR. Adult rat retinal ganglion cells and glia can be printed by piezoelectric inkjet printing. Biofabrication. 2013;**6**(1):015001

Molecular Basis of Neurodegeneration: Lessons from Alzheimer's and Parkinson's Diseases

Juan M. Zolezzi, Sussy Bastías-Candia and
Nibaldo C. Inestrosa

Additional information is available at the end of the chapter

http://dx.doi.org/10.5772/intechopen.81270

Abstract

Alzheimer's disease (AD) and Parkinson's disease (PD) constitute the main causes of dementia worldwide and the major health threats to elderly people. Moreover, with the ageing of the global population, neurodegenerative disorders, such as AD and PD, constitute a major public health issue. Regrettably, significant advances regarding the molecular aspects of these diseases have not yet been translated into real improvements in AD/PD therapeutics. In this regard, both AD and PD are highly complex and involve critical molecular events governing the establishment and progression of each disease. Moreover, molecular alterations trigger pathophysiological cascades involving the immune/inflammatory response, oxidative stress, and mitochondrial dysfunction, among others, ultimately leading to neuronal death. Similarly, these alterations also affect glial cells and brain vasculature, which contribute directly to the progression of these disorders. Accordingly, the present paper aims to summarise the main molecular elements related to AD and PD as well as the pathophysiological implications of such alterations to improve our understanding of the cellular and molecular responses observed during neurodegeneration. We believe that providing a more comprehensive view of the pathophysiological cascade, including neurons and glial cells, might prompt researchers to widen neurodegenerative disorder research and therapeutic approaches.

Keywords: ageing, Alzheimer's, Parkinson's, amyloid-β, α-synuclein, neuroinflammation, oxidative stress, mitochondrial dysfunction

1. Brief introduction to ageing

Undoubtedly, the increased life expectancy of the global population constitutes a major achievement of the modern world. However, it has also opened a gate for the development of age-related conditions that are far from completely understood. In this regard, age-related diseases, particularly neurodegenerative disorders, currently constitute a public health focal point. Accordingly, in recent years, much attention has been focused on understanding both the physiology of ageing and the critical events driving pathological ageing with the subsequent development of different age-related disorders, such as Alzheimer's disease (AD) and Parkinson's disease (PD) [1].

In this regard, ageing constitutes a natural, highly complex process that involves the progressive decay of several biological systems. Moreover, genetic and epigenetic heterogeneity introduces variation in the ageing process from one individual to another [2, 3]. In addition, an increased lifespan implies longer exposure to environmental pollutants that able to interact and modify different biological molecules, including DNA, not only affecting the functionality but also favouring the insurgence of several chronic degenerative disorders (http://www.iarc.fr). Indeed, an altered DNA repair system, systemic and cellular redox imbalance related to mitochondrial dysfunction, sustained pro-inflammatory conditions and impaired immune system functionality are some of the several age-compromised homeostatic systems that can be at the root of pathological changes observed during ageing. Relevantly, and as occurs in other chronic degenerative processes, the breakdown of the homeostatic control and the verification of these alterations seem to depend not only on the impairment of one of the compromised systems but also on the concomitant failure of and crosstalk among others.

As an example, it can be noted that although a reduced methylation status has been recognised as a common condition of the aged genome, the promoter hypermethylation of some genes, with subsequent gene silencing, has also been described [2, 4–7]. The promoters of MutL homologue 1 (MLH1) and MutS homologue 2 (MSH2), both part of the DNA mismatch repair system (MMR), have been reported to be hypermethylated due to arsenic exposure, suggesting an epigenetic-induced DNA MMR impairment that will increase the susceptibility of aged subjects to DNA damage [8]. Whether additional environmental pollutants or inner cellular metabolism end-products can modify the epigenetic control of such relevant mechanisms is an open question [9]. It is important to highlight that both MLH1 and MSH2 are related to the control of the impact that oxidative damage causes on DNA, and both have been observed to decrease during ageing [10]. Concomitantly, and in accordance with Harman's free radical theory [11], the redox balance has been well characterised in aged subjects, indicating that along with the age-related increased production of reactive oxygen and nitrogen species (ROS/RNS), mainly due to mitochondrial failure, the capability of different tissues, including the brain, to buffer ROS/RNS is diminished, as indicated by an increased oxidative status in older subjects [12, 13]. Indeed, the activity of the main ROS/RNS scavengers, including superoxide dismutase (SOD), catalase (CAT), glutathione (GSH) and glutathione peroxidase (GPx), has been demonstrated to decay with ageing, favouring ROS/RNS-related damage, such as lipid peroxidation, protein denaturation and DNA mutations [14, 15]. Moreover, mitochondrial dysfunction, which also constitutes a key element in ageing, is considered one of the major components of the neurodegenerative process observed in both AD and PD. Importantly, beyond the energy impairment, mitochondrial alterations contribute significantly to the increased production of ROS/RNS, increasing the oxidative pressure on the redox equilibrium (**Figure 1**).

On the other hand, it has been well established that chronic exposure to increased levels of pro-oxidant species leads to the concurrent activation of the immune system and triggering of the inflammatory cascade, both further sustained by the release of several pro-inflammatory mediators, such as several interleukins (IL-1, IL-6, IL-8) and interferon-γ (IFN-γ) [16–19]. Moreover, inflammation and the immune response both involve nuclear factor κb (NFκb), a common point that crosslinks both responses. While toll-like receptors (TLRs), which are activated by different subcellular molecular components (damage-associated molecular patterns, DAMPs), signal through NFκb to release several pro-inflammatory cytokines, leading to activation of the immune response, the very same NFκb constitutes an oxidative stress sensor, connecting the increased levels of ROS/RNS with activation of the inflammatory cascade [20, 21]. Additionally, it must be considered that immunocompetence is usually compromised in aged individuals, and several authors have shown that this decay is closely linked to the altered epigenetic control of several immune-related genes [22–24]. Altogether, this evidence suggests that the difference between "normal" and pathological ageing lies in the subtle equilibrium of different homeostatic

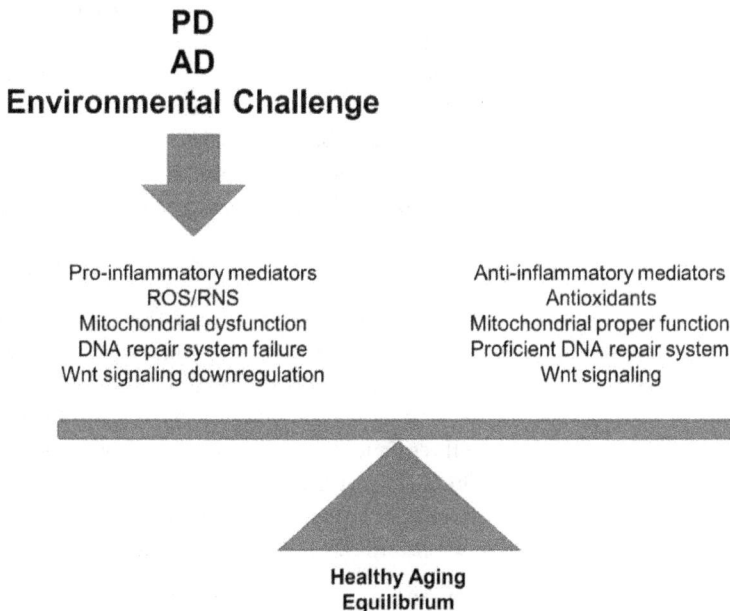

Figure 1. Homeostatic balance against pathological ageing, Alzheimer's disease (AD) and Parkinson's disease (PD). The delicate balance that sustains healthy ageing can be broken under several conditions. Environmental challenges, pathological processes, such as AD and PD, or ageing itself might introduce further pressure in different homeostatic systems, including the immune and redox systems. Moreover, the complex network of molecular alterations, organelle dysfunction and cellular signalling, among others, increases the difficulty of properly addressing the cloudy edge between healthy ageing, pathological ageing and age-related disorders.

systems that can become imbalanced with any additional external/internal stimulus, leading to failure of biological systems and the development of diverse pathological hallmarks.

In the following sections, we will summarise the most relevant aspects of AD and PD and the key elements of each pathophysiological process in the context of the delicate balance of an aged system.

2. Molecular event-driven neurodegeneration: lessons from AD and PD

AD and PD constitute the two most common age-related neurodegenerative disorders [1, 25], and their prevalence is expected to increase together with the ageing of the human population [1]. Although they are different entities, both disorders share some similarities regarding pathophysiological processes (**Figure 2**).

2.1. Alzheimer's disease

In general terms, AD compromises patient memory and cognitive performance. Initially manifesting as mood instability, the clinical scenario progresses from the compromise of short-term memory to the loss of long-term memory. As superior functions are lost, patients become absolutely dependent on a caregiver to complete even the most elementary tasks. Atrophy of the frontal cortex, limbic area and hippocampus due to neuronal death are the basis of these clinical alterations. Histopathologically, AD' shows the extracellular accumulation of amyloid β (Aβ) plaques and the intraneuronal formation of neurofibrillary tangles (NFTs) composed of hyperphosphorylated tau protein [26]. However, even when these molecular events are considered the hallmarks of AD, these alterations are accompanied by an increased oxidative stress status, mitochondrial dysfunction and a chronic inflammatory response, among others, which ultimately serve to explain the synaptic damage, neuronal loss and neuronal circuitry breakdown [26, 27].

Relevantly, although AD constitutes an age-related disorder, an early onset presentation linked to the genetic background should not be omitted. In this regard, while late-onset AD (LOAD) is associated with patients over 65 years old, familial or early-onset AD (EOAD) appears before this threshold, with cases reported as soon as 30 years old. Of course, in EOAD, there is a relevant genetic background in at least three genes (amyloid precursor protein, *APP*; presenilin 1, *PSEN1*; and presenilin 2, *PSEN2*). On the other hand, in the case of LOAD, age and lifestyle are considered to be the main causative factors. Importantly, the apolipoprotein E epsilon 4 (ApoEε4) allele has been identified as a relevant risk factor for both presentation forms [28].

Independent of the presentation form, and as noted previously, Aβ deposition and NFT formation constitute the key molecular features of AD. Moreover, considering that each of the additional pathological alterations often observed during progression of the pathological process can be derived from each of these two hallmarks, each of them has led to the development of individual hypotheses. Although the crosstalk between the amyloid and tau hypotheses is evident, it must be noted that the scientific community has not yet agreed on which one encompasses the whole spectrum of the disease, and the aetiological trigger of the pathological molecular cascade remains unknown.

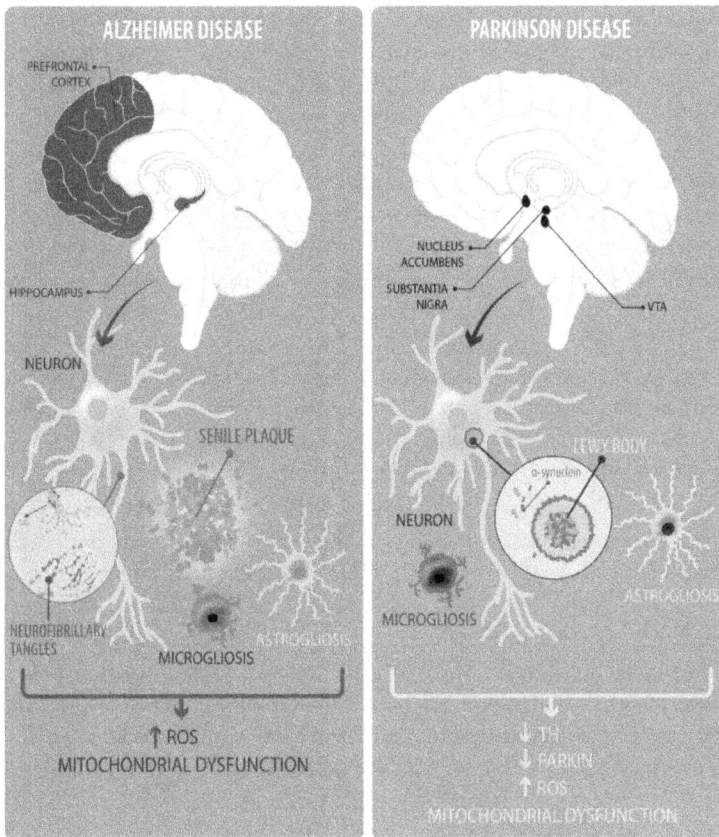

Figure 2. Alzheimer's disease (AD) and Parkinson's disease (PD). Pathological milieu overview. AD and PD are highly complex disorders. In both cases, in addition to the molecular hallmarks, cellular alterations are verified. Although several risk factors have been identified, the aetiology of both disorders is still unknown. AD is characterised by neuronal loss, mainly in the hippocampus. The pathognomonic feature of AD is the deposition of amyloid-β aggregates (senile plaques) and the formation of neurofibrillary tangles composed of hyperphosphorylated tau protein. These molecular alterations not only affect neurons but also induce microglial and astrocytic activation, leading to the release of several pro-inflammatory mediators. Additionally, cellular and molecular events will cause an increased production of reactive oxygen/nitrogen species, which will further damage the surrounding neurons and activate the surrounding glial cells, perpetuating the inflammatory response. In contrast, PD is characterised by the loss of dopaminergic circuitry beginning at the basal forebrain (substantia nigra pars compacta (SNpc), nucleus accumbens and ventral tegmental area (VTA)) and spreading to the striatum. The molecular hallmark of PD is the formation of Lewy bodies and neurites, which are composed of aggregated α-synuclein (SNCA), causing severe cellular stress affecting the cytoskeleton, neuronal trafficking and the synthesis of dopamine because of the direct inhibition of tyrosine hydroxylase (TH). SCNA can be exocytosed, causing it to be internalised by astrocytes, where it can further aggregate. Similarly, it will cause microglial activation. Neurons, astrocytes and microglia release pro-inflammatory mediators as well as ROS/RNS. A common feature of both disorders is mitochondrial dysfunction, which can be due to the pathological process or the result of the homeostatic imbalance verified during abnormal ageing.

Even with several additional hypotheses having been developed since the first description of AD by Dr. Alois Alzheimer, including the "cholinergic hypothesis" [29], from our limited expertise in the field, we approach AD considering the increased production and subsequent accumulation of Aβ within the brain as the starting point. Indeed, synaptic failure, mitochondrial dysfunction, tau hyperphosphorylation, glial activation and neuronal death, among others, can be explained by the Aβ dynamics [27, 30]. According to this theory, AD results from the increased levels of Aβ, a 37- to 49-amino acid peptide derived from the proteolytic processing of APP, because of an unbalanced production/clearance rate [31–33]. In this regard, under the AD scenario, the non-amyloidogenic processing of APP, carried out by the alpha (α) and gamma (γ) secretases, which leads to the release of soluble APPα (sAPPα) and the p3 fragment, is overwhelmed by amyloidogenic processing, with beta (β) secretase (BACE1) as the main player, leading to an increased release of the neurotoxic Aβ peptide [30, 33]. On the other hand, under balanced physiological conditions, Aβ is cleared to the blood stream and cerebrospinal fluid (CSF), with the involvement of ApoE, the Aβ chaperone [30, 31], through several transporter proteins, including members of the ATP-binding cassette family of transporters, such as ABCB1, ABCC2 and ABCG4, and the low-density lipoprotein receptor-related protein/ApoE receptor (LRP/APOER), the main receptor responsible for Aβ clearance through the blood-brain barrier (BBB) [30, 34–36]. ApoE deficiency/incompetence (ApoEε4), altered Aβ-related transporter expression, choroid plexus and BBB damage will impair Aβ clearance, increasing brain Aβ levels. Additionally, the reduced activity of Aβ-degrading enzymes, such as disintegrin and metalloproteases (ADAM 9, 10 and 17A) and neprilysin, will further contribute to its accumulation within the brain [32, 33, 37–40]. At this point, the increased levels of Aβ will favour its self-aggregation, leading to the formation of different Aβ species, such as oligomers, fibrils and/or even larger aggregates, such as plaques [26, 29]. Moreover, the presence of APP together with its proteolytic machinery within the subcellular compartments, such as the Golgi and endoplasmic reticulum (ER), as well as the presence of Aβ peptide in the mitochondria, suggests that the intracellular APP dynamics can also be part of the pathological scenario along with the extracellular accumulation of Aβ peptide. Indeed, it has been demonstrated that in the presence of high levels of Aβ, the peptide can enter the cell through the presynapticα 7 nicotinic acetylcholine receptor and that this influx could be the basis for tau hyperphosphorylation, thereby causing neurite atrophy and synapse failure [30].

2.2. Parkinson's disease

PD is the second most common neurodegenerative disorder and can be classified as a synucleinopathy. It is characterised by failure of the dopaminergic circuitry because of the loss of dopaminergic neurons of the substantia nigra pars compacta (SNpc). Histopathologically, PD shows neuronal inclusions of aggregated α-synuclein (SNCA) protein in both the cell soma and neurites, forming Lewy bodies and neurites [25]. Although the effects of the loss of dopaminergic neurons help to explain the symptomatology, mainly associated with motor compromise, the mechanisms by which SNCA aggregates in relation to the whole molecular and clinical picture have remained elusive. Ranging from non-motor symptoms, including hyposmia and sleep disturbances, PD progresses to bradykinesia and rigidity and can be accompanied by impairments in memory, mainly prospective memory [25, 41, 42].

Similar to AD, genetic background also accounts for a small proportion of PD cases worldwide. β-Glucocerebrosidase (GBA), leucine-rich repeat kinase 2 (LRRK2), SNCA, parkin (PRKN), protein/nucleic acid deglycase (DJ1) and phosphatase and tensin homologue (PTEN)-induced putative kinase 1 (PINK1) have been recognised as the most relevant genes associated with PD presentation [25, 43]. On the other hand, sporadic PD has been related to age and lifestyle, mainly regarding exposure to different types of chemicals, including agrochemicals and drugs [25, 44]. With the increase in life expectancy, the global PD prevalence is expected to double over the next decade.

As noted previously, independent of the presentation form, SNCA aggregates constitute the pathological hallmark of PD. In this regard, SNCA corresponds to a monomeric 140-amino acid protein localised at the presynaptic terminal, which is thought to be involved in the recycling of synaptic vesicle pools [45–47]. Although 50% of the protein can be found at the cytosolic level within the terminals, the remaining SNCA is associated with the membrane of both vesicles and early endosomes. Indeed, SNCA has been described as a chaperone protein of the soluble N-ethylmaleimide-sensitive factor attachment protein receptor (SNARE) proteins [48]. However, the mechanisms related to the interaction of SNCA with SNARE or additional presynaptic proteins, such as Piccolo/Bassoon or Rab, and its function in regulating the dynamics of the synaptic terminal are still unknown [43, 49, 50]. Under pathological conditions, SNCA changes from a monomeric membrane-associated protein to an unbound monomer capable of forming β-sheet aggregates, which ultimately will form SNCA amyloid fibrils [50–52]. Moreover, SNCA can not only interfere with tyrosine hydroxylase, the dopamine synthesis enzyme, affecting both its expression and activity [53], but also interact with the dopamine transporter (DAT) [54]. At this point, and considering the altered synaptic vesicle dynamics, the dopaminergic synapse is severely compromised, constituting the basis of the PD synaptopathy. Additionally, similar to AD, this initial molecular event can be related to the additional features observed during the pathological process, including mitochondrial dysfunction, increased oxidative stress, and neuroinflammation.

3. Pathophysiological cascade in AD and PD

3.1. Inflammation and the CNS

Immunocompetence constitutes a fundamental feature for ensuring the preservation of any living organism. The rapid and coordinated elimination of potentially harmful elements is critical to maintain organism homeostasis and prevent irreversible damage to biological systems. In this regard, the innate and adaptive immune systems constitute the two subsystems that able to detect and induce a primary unspecific response to pathogens, coordinate a secondary response and develop an immune memory, the hallmark of adaptive immunity. As the first response element, the innate immune system depends on the effectiveness of several unspecific elements, including physical and chemical barriers, the complement system, the activity of surveillance cells, and inflammation. Through these complementary elements, a fundamental physiological process is triggered to constrain the insult and repair the damage. In general, whether because of a pathogen, toxic and/or damaged-cell end-products, the cellular microenvironment will change, leading to the activation of immunocompetent cells and causing the release of pro- and anti-inflammatory cytokines, such as tumour necrosis factor 1α (TNF-1α), interleukins (IL-1, IL-8, IL-10), interferon γ (INF-γ) and transforming growth factor 1 (TGF-1), to orchestrate a coordinated response against the primary insult, limiting its damage [55, 56]. Importantly, to appropriately answer signals of harm/damage, surveillance cells need to express several types of receptors. Moreover, considering that harm/damage signals can be both exogenous, such as those from bacteria and viruses, and endogenous, such as those from DNA or ATP, these receptors should be able to interact with a wide range of these elements. Among the latter, TLRs constitute a key element of the innate immune response related to sterile inflammatory pathological processes, such as AD and PD. It is important to highlight that even when it was initially considered an immune-privileged system, because of its high specialisation and partial isolation from the rest of the organism, the central nervous system (CNS) is able to generate full-range immune responses. In this context, microglia and astrocytes are responsible for immune surveillance in the CNS, with microglia being the only immune-derived cells within the brain. Due to the critical role of the brain microenvironment, evidence suggests that the inflammatory response is tightly controlled to prevent the detrimental effects of an exacerbated process. Indeed, it has been determined that the brain parenchyma constitutes an anti-inflammatory environment with relevant levels of TGF and IL-10 [57, 58].

3.2. TLR-mediated neuroinflammatory response

TLRs are able to detect DAMPs, which are subcellular components, such as ATP, released into the extracellular media reflecting cell damage. Several members of the TLR family have been described and can be expressed at the plasma membrane, such as TLRs 1, 2, 4, 5, and 6, or in association with endosomes, such as TLRs 3, 7, 8, and 9. Importantly, TLRs are expressed by brain cells, including astrocytes, microglia, neurons and oligodendrocytes, with microglia and neurons expressing all TLR subtypes and astrocytes expressing a more limited repertoire, including TLR2, TLR3, TLR4, TLR9 and TLR11 [59, 60]. Briefly, the TLR-mediated modulation of the inflammatory response begins with the recruitment of myeloid differentiation factor 88 (MyD88), causing activation of the IL-1 receptor-associated kinase (IRAK) family of proteins. IRAK activates TNF receptor-associated factor 6 (TRAF6), causing the recruitment of TGF-β-activated kinase 1 (TAK1). TAK1, along with TAK1-binding proteins (TABs), will activate the IKK complex, causing phosphorylation of the IkB factor and the subsequent release of NF-kB to translocate into the nucleus, leading to the expression of NF-kB-related inflammatory genes. Importantly, TLRs 3 and 4 can also signal via a secondary TIR-containing adaptor inducing an IFN-β (TRIF)-mediated pathway. Additionally, in the latter case, NF-kB will be released, but IFN-β will be produced because of the phosphorylation of IFN regulatory factors 3 and 7 (IRF3–7) via IKKe/TANK-binding kinase 1 (TBK1). Independent of the cascade triggered through TLRs, the final outcome will be the production and release of cytokines, chemokines, complement proteins and enzymes, including several members of the IL family, such as IL-1, IL-6, IL-10, IL-11, and IL-12, as well as TNF, TGF, IFN, CCL2, CCL5, CXCL8 and CXCL10 [59–62]. An additional clue about the necessity of tightly controlling this process within a highly specialised organ, such as the brain, emerges from the property of these molecules to further activate TLRs, a situation that can lead to re-activation of the inflammatory cascade and a state of chronic inflammation.

In this regard, the inflammatory component of AD and PD has been demonstrated to be fundamental for both pathological processes. Moreover, it has been shown that both Aβ and SNCA can induce direct activation of the inflammatory response and that their sustained accumulation and aggregation lead to the genesis of a pro-inflammatory environment [21, 63,

64]. Indeed, during the recent year, the modulation and control of the inflammatory cascade have emerged as target elements of future therapeutic interventions aimed at improving AD and PD outcomes [34, 64, 65].

3.2.1. TLRs and Aβ peptide in AD

Evidence indicates that TLR2 and TLR4 are able to react with Aβ, leading to the release of several pro-inflammatory mediators, such as IL-1β, IL-6, IL-12, TNF-α, cyclooxygenase 2 (COX2) and inducible nitric oxide synthase (iNOS) [66]. As noted previously, such receptors are expressed by different cell types present in the brain, suggesting both the whole-brain commitment to the inflammatory response and the potential contribution of all these cells to the further release of pro-inflammatory mediators. In this regard, of the most relevance is the self-perpetuation of the inflammatory cycle induced by the continuous release of these molecules. Some of the pro-inflammatory cytokines, such as IL-6, which can be produced as part of the response to the initial insult (Aβ), can also be a consequence of the secondary effect induced by other cytokines, such as IL-1β [67]. Thus, if this response is not controlled, the environment can be perfectly suited to a sustained pro-inflammatory status that will over-whelm homeostatic mechanisms and damage the surrounding tissue.

Furthermore, Aβ can trigger additional molecular events within neurons. Beyond its pro-inflammatory effects, it has been demonstrated that Aβ can induce the hyperphosphoryla-tion of tau protein, which will alter the neuronal cytoskeleton, ultimately leading to neuronal apoptosis with the release of further DAMPs [26, 27, 29, 35]. Evidently, this situation can also promote TLR activation, contributing to perpetuation of the inflammatory cycle. Similarly, astrocytes, which express a more limited repertoire of TLRs, are also fundamental for ade-quate Aβ metabolism. In the case of AD, astrocytes are responsible for the release of ApoE, the Aβ chaperone protein necessary for its removal from the brain. In this context, defective astro-cytes, such as inflammatory-challenged astrocytes, or ApoE-related genetic conditions, such as the ApoEε4 allele, can lead to impaired ApoE activity, causing an increase in the Aβ level [31]. Again, these astrocyte-related conditions can compromise the brain's ability to resolve the inflammatory process and further contribute to enhancing a detrimental inflammatory response. In contrast, microglia, as the only representative of the immune system within the brain parenchyma, are the main cells responsible for surveying and initiating the immune response against exogenous and endogenous insults, acting as the macrophages of the brain. Microglia develop a close interaction with neurons through microglial chemokine (C-X-C motif) receptor 1 (CXCR1) and CD200L, with neuronal CX3CL1 and CD200, respectively [68, 69]. In the absence of a challenging stimulus, microglia remain in a non-inflammatory or "resting" state. However, when inflammatory signals, such as the loss of neuronal contact or DAMPs, are detected, microglia undergo morphological and physiological changes leading to an inflammatory or "activated" state. Among the several receptors expressed by microglia, TLRs 1–9 and the co-receptor CD14 are the most important for its activation [21]. Although it has been demonstrated that Aβ directly activates TLR2 and TLR4, it has recently been shown that additional elements are involved in the activity of microglia in response to aggregated forms of Aβ. Complement receptor 1 (CR1), cluster of differentiation 33 (CD33) and triggering receptor expressed on myeloid cells 2 (TREM2) have proven to be necessary for the successful phagocytosis of Aβ [70–72]. Moreover, it has been suggested that TREM2 acts as a receptor for Aβ, thereby modulating the microglial inflammatory response [73]. The relevance of the functions related to TREM2 activity has led us to consider its proteolytic products (soluble TREM2) as potential biomarkers for AD, mainly because sTREM2 levels have been reported to be elevated in the plasma and CSF of AD patients [73–75]. The precise impact of such findings is just emerging, and some discrepancies have already been identified regarding which should be the appropriate approach to a TREM2-related intervention [76, 77].

3.2.2. TLRs and SNCA in PD

Similar to Aβ, different research groups have shown that SNCA induces the inflammatory response through a TLR2- and TLR4-mediated mechanism, leading to TNF-α, IL-6 and CXCL1 expression via the MyD88-NF-kB pathway [78–80]. Interestingly, it has been demonstrated that while monomeric SNCA activates TLR2, the oligomeric forms tend to activate TLR4 [81]. Complimentarily, a relevant issue has emerged from recent research which has demonstrated that inflammation itself, through a caspase-mediated mechanism, can favour the aggregation of SNCA [51, 52]. This latter finding further support the idea of a self-sustained cycle which amplifies the initial damage exerted by the SNCA and contributes to the progression of the pathology. However, beyond the TLR-NF-kB axis and the production of pro-inflammatory mediators, additional aspects should be considered regarding SNCA hallmarks.

Within neurons, aggregated SNCA, whether in the soma or in neurites, will cause cell death with the subsequent release of cellular content, the components of which will release additional DAMPs capable of interacting with additional TLRs [82]. Moreover, it has been demonstrated that SNCA can be exocytosed actively from neurons, incorporated by the surrounding astrocytes, and then further aggregated, causing the formation of inclusion bodies within the new host cells [83]. Considering that the primary function of astrocytes is related to providing metabolic support to neurons and modulating the neurotransmitter metabolism within synapses, the SNCA pathology will not only involve the inflammatory response of astrocytes but will compromise its physiology, enhancing the neuronal network damage verified during PD pathophysiology [84–86]. On the other hand, although microglia will react to SNCA through TLRs, SNCA can also influence the activity of activated microglia against further pro-inflammatory signals, suggesting that SNCA can induce a priming effect on the microglia population, exerting a type of modulation on the strength of the inflammatory response [70, 87]. Thus, in the case of SNCA, this molecule can not only induce/perpetuate a pro-inflammatory status but also lead to an increased susceptibility to any inflammatory process.

3.3. Mitochondrial dysfunction

An additional common feature of both pathologies is the increased production of ROS/RNS. Indeed, an important end point of glial activation is that in response to the initial inflammatory trigger, Aβ in the case of AD and SNCA in PD, astrocytes and microglia will produce not only further inflammatory mediators, such as TNF-α and ILs, but also ROS/RNS [85]. The increased production of ROS and RNS will alter the surrounding microenvironment, and these species will be able to interact with the lipids of the plasma membrane, proteins and nucleic acids of the contiguous cells, ultimately affecting component of the neuronal circuitry, such as synapses, axons and whole cell structures [88–90]. In this context, mitochondrial activity, which is fundamental to sustaining neuronal activity, is one of the major sources of the continuous production of superoxide anions. This highly reactive species, if not neutralised, will severely damage subcellular structures. Under regular conditions, superoxide anions are scavenged as soon as they are produced through hydrogen peroxide formation. However, under altered redox conditions, such as those during ageing, cellular mechanisms to manage both physiological and pathological ROS/RNS production are overwhelmed [12–15]. Thus, AD and PD cause additional pressure on the mitochondria in an already poorly balanced system.

In this regard, both Aβ and SNCA have been demonstrated to be able to alter mitochondria. While Aβ has been found within mitochondria, indicating a direct effect on mitochondrial functionality [91, 92], SNCA can impair mitochondrial function mainly via altered cell trafficking. Indeed, it has recently been suggested that the cytoskeletal alterations induced by SNCA will modulate the localization of dynamin-related protein 1 (Drp1), a key protein related to mitochondrial dynamics and whose malfunction will lead to mitochondrial dysfunction [93, 94]. Complimentarily, Aβ, and probably SNCA, can induce ER stress, leading to the intracellular release of Ca^{2+}, which can increase the mitochondrial challenge, leading to further ROS/RNS production and causing the subsequent activation of classical pro-apoptotic pathways, such as ROS-mediated apoptosis through apoptosis signal-regulated kinase (ASK1) and activation of the B cell lymphoma 2 (BCL2)-beclin 1 (BECN1) complex [91, 92]. It should not be forgotten that ROS/RNS can trigger the inflammatory response in surrounding cells, such as glial cells and neighbouring neurons, in a TLR- and DAMP-mediated manner. Moreover, it is possible that prior to the pathological process, these aged individuals have some degree of inflammation, oxidative stress and mitochondrial impairment, which might facilitate the establishment and/or progression of both diseases.

4. Wnt signalling in the context of AD and PD anti-inflammatory therapeutics

Currently, neurodegenerative disorders, especially AD and PD, are considered a major concern in public health because of the ageing of the global population. Although some progress has been made regarding pharmacological strategies, regrettably, no effective therapies are currently available to stop or reverse these pathologies. Among the alternative approaches to overcome such situations, the identification and further modulation of key cellular pathways involved in the pathophysiology of neurodegenerative disorders should not be underestimated. In this regard, even when it is well recognised that inflammation is one of the most relevant features of AD and PD, anti-inflammatory therapies have remained overlooked, although some epidemiological data have suggested a significant effect in terms of risk reduction with the use of some nonsteroidal anti-inflammatory drugs (NSAIDs) [95, 96]. Interestingly, the main effects related to the use of such a family of drugs have been observed prior to the onset of pathology; however, the efficacy of an anti-inflammatory therapy cannot be fully discarded. Indeed, the reasons behind the failure of some clinical trials exploring the beneficial effects of NSAIDs in AD and PD have not been properly addressed [97]. Moreover, a quick search of scientific databases, such as PubMed, will return over 3000 and 1000 entries for AD and PD, respectively, when both "anti-inflammatory therapy" and "AD/PD" are used as search terms. This issue not only reinforces the fact that inflammation is a key element of both pathologies but also indicates that the inflammatory cascade is closely related to several signalling pathways that have been linked to the pathophysiology of these diseases. Regrettably, our understanding of these mechanisms is incomplete, limiting our capacity to properly address and exploit such relationships.

In this regard, over several decades, our laboratory has been working on Wnt signalling, a master cellular pathway involved in both physiological and pathological conditions. The activity of Wnt signalling varies with ageing depending on the tissue [98]. Specifically, in the brain, an overall downregulation of the Wnt pathway is observed, suggesting that some of the impairments associated with age might be mediated by this Wnt decay [98, 99]. Accordingly, this situation suggests that the rescuing of its activity might be a promising strategy to prevent and alleviate some of the pathological features of AD and PD.

4.1. Wnt signalling pathway

From the initial steps during embryogenesis to the less explored adult neurogenesis, the Wnt pathway constitutes the core molecular signalling pathway of cellular physiology. Its relevance is demonstrated by the evolutionary conservation of this system among different species, and its potentialities are cross-linked with the outcome of different neurodegenerative disorders, including AD and PD [100, 101].

The Wnt pathway is commonly divided into two canonical or β-catenin-dependent and non-canonical pathways, with the latter further divided into Wnt/Ca^{++} and planar cell polarity (JNK). Briefly, in the canonical pathway, the Wnt ligands bind to Frizzled receptor/low-density lipoprotein receptor-related protein 5/6 (Fz/LRP5/6) and the subsequent activation of Dishevelled. This situation leads to disassembly of the β-catenin destruction complex comprising adenoma polyposis coli (APC), Axin, GSK3β and casein kinase 1 (CK1), leaving β-catenin free to translocate to the nucleus and initiate transcription of the Wnt target genes together with the T-cell factor/lymphoid enhancer factor (TCF/Lef) transcription factor. In the absence of Wnt ligands, the destruction complex remains active, and GSK3b phosphorylates β-catenin, causing its proteasomal degradation. On the other hand, in Wnt/planar cell polarity, the binding of Wnt ligands will induce cytoskeletal rearrangements via JNK-mediated mechanisms; in the Wnt/Ca^{++} pathway, ligand binding induces the release of Ca^{2+} from the ER, causing the activation of several calcium-related proteins, such as protein kinase C (PKC) and calcium/calmodulin-dependent protein kinase (Ca^{2+}/CamKII) [21, 100].

Additionally, the different cascades described for Wnt signalling can interact with several cellular pathways, including the forkhead box O (FOXO), Notch and hypoxia-inducible factor 1 alpha (HIF1α) pathways [93]. Precisely, the wide range of molecular interactions established by Wnt signalling serves to explain how its altered activity can not only favour or directly induce different pathological conditions, including neurodegenerative disorders and cancer, but also act as a relevant player in the ageing process. In this regard, we have recently demonstrated that the loss of Wnt signalling favours the appearance of several pathological markers linked to AD in a wild-type murine model [102]. Moreover, we found that Wnt signalling is involved in the neuronal energy metabolism and that its activation rescues energy imbalance because of improved glucose utilisation [103]. On the other hand, Wnt signalling also plays a relevant role in PD. It has been demonstrated that LRRK2 can interact with several members of the β-catenin destruction complex, including Dvl, Axin, GSK3β and β-catenin [104]. Similarly, PRKN is related to the ubiquitination of β-catenin, playing a direct role in the modulation of this pathway [105]. The relevance of such regulation has prompted some researchers to propose the pharmacological modulation of Wnt signalling as a relevant target in PD [106]. Complimentary to these well-established effects, Wnt signalling has also been linked to modulation and crosstalk within the inflammatory cascade.

4.2. Wnt signalling and the inflammatory pathway

Although it could be considered circumstantial, the inflammatory status and Wnt signalling are inversely correlated during the ageing process; in other words, while the pro-inflammatory status increases with age, Wnt signalling decreases. Of course, additional signalling pathways are impaired during ageing; however, the fact that Wnt is able to modulate the NF-kB pathway strongly suggests that this particular pathway has a direct impact on the immune/inflammatory response observed during the ageing process. Moreover, it should be considered that even when it is well accepted that canonical Wnt signalling has anti-inflammatory activity and the non-canonical pathway exerts a pro-inflammatory effect, these opposing functions can be carried out by the same ligand, such as Wnt5a [21, 101]. This latter finding also suggests that depending on the physiological or pathological status of the biological system, Wnt components can exert different modulatory effects to contribute to the maintenance of system balance. In contrast, inflammation can also modulate Wnt activity. In this regard, TLR activation can downregulate the canonical Wnt signalling pathway. While TLR4 causes the blockade of the Fz-LRP5/6 complex [107], MyD88-mediated TLR activity activates nemo-like kinase (NLK), which interacts with the nuclear β-catenin-TCF/Lef complex. Similarly, MyD88-independent TLR signalling activates IKKe/TBK1, which can directly phosphorylate Akt, leading to GSK3β inhibition and blocking the activity of the β-catenin destruction complex [108–111].

Although evidence demonstrates a close relationship between Wnt signalling and the inflammatory process, our knowledge regarding this issue remains limited. Moreover, the already proven involvement and the critical role that Wnt signalling seems to play in different aspects of physiological and pathological cellular mechanisms certainly indicate that this pathway needs to be investigated deeply to properly assess the effects of finely modulating Wnt signalling, including its potentially beneficial effects in the context of the inflammatory response. In this regard, part of our work suggests that lithium and andrographolide, both well-established canonical Wnt agonists that act via GSK3β inhibition, can play a relevant role not only under pathological conditions but also as exogenous support of a healthy ageing process by reducing several markers of unhealthy conditions, including neuroinflammation [112].

5. Final considerations

According to the available evidence, ageing constitutes a vulnerable stage for cell fate mainly because of the delicate balance of several molecular conditions. Under these conditions, any additional challenge to any homeostatic system can trigger the breakdown of such equilibrium, leading to the manifestation of pathological processes, such as neurodegenerative disorders. AD and PD, the first and second most prevalent age-related diseases, can be favoured by a spontaneous imbalance in the homeostatic system and, once initiated, further contribute to increasing the homeostatic imbalance. A complex network of molecular alterations, organelle dysfunction and cellular signalling, among others, increases the difficulty of properly addressing the cloudy edge between healthy ageing, pathological ageing and age-related disorders. However, neuroinflammation and the perpetuation of a chronic pro-inflammatory status have emerged as a central axis connecting all these conditions. Although our knowledge regarding the inflammatory process has increased during years, the intricate molecular network that drives the final inflammatory response is still incomplete. In this regard, Wnt signalling, which has been demonstrated to be a relevant player in ageing and age-related disorders, such as AD and PD, should also be considered among the potentially relevant molecular pathways that could be involved in the modulation of the inflammatory process. Moreover, the still limited information regarding the Wnt-inflammatory response crosstalk already suggests interesting potentialities of an anti-inflammatory intervention based on the modulation of Wnt signalling. On the other hand, based on our research and considering the age-related changes in Wnt activity, it is possible to suggest that Wnt signalling can also be an interesting target to support physiological ageing.

Funding

This work was funded by Basal Center of Excellence in Science and Technology CONICYT PIA/BASAL PFB 12 (CONICYT-PFB12/2007) to NCI and by FONDECYT N° 11170212 to SBC.

Author details

Juan M. Zolezzi[1], Sussy Bastías-Candia[1] and Nibaldo C. Inestrosa[1,2,3*]

*Address all correspondence to: ninestrosa@bio.puc.cl

1 Centro de Envejecimiento y Regeneración (CARE), Departamento de Biología Celular y Molecular, Facultad de Ciencias Biológicas, Pontificia Universidad Católica de Chile, Santiago, Chile

2 Centre for Healthy Brain Ageing, School of Psychiatry, Faculty of Medicine, University of New South Wales, Sydney, Australia

3 Centro de Excelencia en Biomedicina de Magallanes (CEBIMA), Universidad de Magallanes, Punta Arenas, Chile

References

[1] Alzheimer's Disease International. World Alzheimer Report. 2016. Available from: https://www.alz.co.uk/research/world-report [Accessed: 2017-11-20]

[2] Ashapkin VV, Kutueva LI, Vanyushin BF. Aging as an epigenetic phenomenon. Current Genomics. 2017;**18**:385-407. DOI: 10.2174/1389202918666170412112130

[3] Masser DR, Hadad N, Porter HL, Mangold CA, Unnikrishnan A, Ford MM, et al. Sexually divergent DNA methylation patterns with hippocampal aging. Aging Cell. 2017;**16**:1342-1352. DOI: 10.1111/acel.12681

[4] Hadad N, Unnikrishnan A, Jackson JA, Masser DR, Otalora L, Stanford DR, et al. Caloric restriction mitigates age-associated hippocampal differential CG and non-CG methylation. Neurobiology of Aging. 2018;**67**:53-66. DOI: 10.1016/j.neurobiolaging.2018.03.009

[5] Wezyk M, Spólnicka M, Pośpiech E, Pepłońska B, Zbieć-Piekarska R, Ilkowski J, et al. Hypermethylation of TRIM59 and KLF14 influences cell death signaling in familial Alzheimer's disease. Oxidative Medicine and Cellular Longevity. 2018;**2018**:6918797. DOI: 10.1155/2018/6918797

[6] Lardenoije R, van den Hove DLA, Havermans M, van Casteren A, Le KX, Palmour R, et al. Age-related epigenetic changes in hippocampal subregions of four animal models of Alzheimer's disease. Molecular and Cellular Neurosciences. 2018;**86**:1-15. DOI: 10.1016/j.mcn.2017.11.002

[7] Berson A, Nativio R, Berger SL, Bonini NM. Epigenetic regulation in neurodegenerative diseases. Trends in Neurosciences. 2018;**S0166-2236**:30133-30134. DOI: 10.1016/j.tins.2018.05.005

[8] Bhattacharjee P, Sanyal T, Bhattacharjee S, Bhattacharjee P. Epigenetic alteration of mismatch repair genes in the population chronically exposed to arsenic in West Bengal, India. Environmental Research. 2018;**163**:289-296. DOI: 10.1016/j.envres.2018.01.002

[9] Skinner AM, Turker MS. Oxidative mutagenesis, mismatch repair, and aging. Science of Aging Knowledge Environment. 2005;**2005**:re3. DOI: 10.1126/sageke.2005.9.re3

[10] Conde-Pérezprina JC, León-Galván MÁ, Konigsberg M. DNA mismatch repair system: Repercussions in cellular homeostasis and relationship with aging. Oxidative Medicine and Cellular Longevity. 2012;**2012**:728430. DOI: 10.1155/2012/728430

[11] Harman D. Aging: A theory based on free radical and radiation chemistry. Journal of Gerontology. 1956;**11**:298-300

[12] Lushchak VI. Free radicals, reactive oxygen species, oxidative stress and its classification. Chemico-Biological Interactions. 2014;**224**:164-175. DOI: 10.1016/j.cbi.2014.10.016

[13] Garaschuk O, Semchyshyn HM, Lushchak VI. Healthy brain aging: Interplay between reactive species, inflammation and energy supply. Ageing Research Reviews. 2018;**43**:26-45. DOI: 10.1016/j.arr.2018.02.003

[14] Samarghandian S, Azimi-Nezhad M, Samini F. Preventive effect of safranal against oxidative damage in aged male rat brain. Experimental Animals. 2015;**64**:65-71. DOI: 10.1538/expanim.14-0027

[15] Liu C, Li X, Lu B. The Immp2l mutation causes age-dependent degeneration of cerebellar granule neurons prevented by antioxidant treatment. Aging Cell. 2016;**15**:167-176. DOI: 10.1111/acel.12426

[16] Meier B, Radeke HH, Selle S, Raspe HH, Sies H, Resch K, et al. Human fibroblasts release reactive oxygen species in response to treatment with synovial fluids from patients suffering from arthritis. Free Radical Research Communications. 1990;**8**:149-160. DOI: 10.3109/10715769009087988

[17] Roberts RA, Smith RA, Safe S, Szabo C, Tjalkens RB, Robertson FM. Toxicological and pathophysiological roles of reactive oxygen and nitrogen species. Toxicology. 2010;**276**:85-94. DOI: 10.1016/j.tox.2010.07.009

[18] Dandekar A, Mendez R, Zhang K. Cross talk between ER stress, oxidative stress, and inflammation in health and disease. Methods in Molecular Biology. 2015;**1292**:205-214. DOI: 10.1007/978-1-4939-2522-3_15

[19] Franceschi C, Garagnani P, Vitale G, Capri M, Salvioli S. Inflammaging and 'Garb-aging'. Trends in Endocrinology and Metabolism. 2017;**28**:199-212. DOI: 10.1016/j.tem.2016.09.005

[20] Muriach M, Flores-Bellver M, Romero FJ, Barcia JM. Diabetes and the brain: Oxidative stress, inflammation, and autophagy. Oxidative Medicine and Cellular Longevity. 2014;**2014**:102158. DOI: 10.1155/2014/102158

[21] Zolezzi JM, Inestrosa NC. Wnt/TLR dialog in neuroinflammation, relevance in Alzheimer's disease. Frontiers in Immunology. 2017;**8**:187. DOI: 10.3389/fimmu.2017.00187

[22] Wei L, Liu B, Tuo J, Shen D, Chen P, Li Z, et al. Hypomethylation of IL17RC promoter associates with age-related macular degeneration. Cell Reports. 2012;**2**:1151-1158. DOI: 10.1016/j.celrep.2012.10.013

[23] Marttila S, Kananen L, Hayrynen S, Jylhava J, Nevalainen T, Hervonen A, et al. Ageing-associated changes in the human DNA methylome: Genomic locations and effects on gene expression. BMC Genomics. 2015;**16**:179. DOI: 10.1186/s12864-015-1381-z

[24] Zhao M, Qin J, Yin H, Tan Y, Liao W, Liu Q, et al. Distinct epigenomes in CD4+ T cells of newborns, middle-ages and centenarians. Scientific Reports. 2016;**6**:38411. DOI: 10.1038/srep38411

[25] Kalia LV, Lang AE. Parkinson's disease. Lancet. 2015;**386**:896-912. DOI: 10.1016/S0140-6736(14)61393-3

[26] Selkoe DJ. Alzheimer's disease. Cold Spring Harbor Perspectives in Biology. 2011;**3**: a004457. DOI: 10.1101/cshperspect.a004457

[27] Selkoe DJ, Hardy J. The amyloid hypothesis of Alzheimer's disease at 25 years. EMBO Molecular Medicine. 2016;**8**:595-608. DOI: 10.15252/emmm.201606210

[28] Bird TD. Early-onset familial Alzheimer disease. In: Pagon RA, Adam MP, Ardinger HH, et al., editors. Genes Reviews. Seattle (WA): University of Washington, Seattle: 1993-2017

[29] Carvajal FJ, Inestrosa NC. Interactions of AChE with Aβ aggregates in Alzheimer's brain: Therapeutic relevance of IDN 5706. Frontiers in Molecular Neuroscience. 2011;**4**:19. DOI: 10.3389/fnmol.2011.00019

[30] Zolezzi JM, Bastías-Candia S, Santos MJ, Inestrosa NC. Alzheimer's disease: Relevant molecular and physiopathological events affecting amyloid-β brain balance and the putative role of PPARs. Frontiers in Aging Neuroscience. 2014;**6**:176. DOI: 10.3389/fnagi.2014.00176

[31] Cramer PE, Cirrito JR, Wesson DW, Lee CY, Karlo JC, Zinn AE, et al. ApoE-directed therapeutics rapidly clear β-amyloid and reverse deficits in AD mouse models. Science. 2012;**335**:1503-1506. DOI: 10.1126/science.1217697

[32] Singh I, Sagare AP, Coma M, Perlmutter D, Gelein R, Bell RD, et al. Low levels of copper disrupt brain amyloid-β homeostasis by altering its production and clearance. Proceedings of the National Academy of Sciences of the United States of America. 2013;**110**:14771-14776. DOI: 10.1073/pnas.1302212110

[33] Yan R, Vassar R. Targeting the β secretase BACE1 for Alzheimer's disease therapy. Lancet Neurology. 2014;**13**:319-329. DOI: 10.1016/S1474-4422(13) 70276-X

[34] Zolezzi JM, Inestrosa NC. Peroxisome proliferator-activated receptors and Alzheimer's disease: Hitting the blood-brain barrier. Molecular Neurobiology. 2013;**48**:438-451. DOI: 10.1007/s12035-013-8435-5

[35] Zlokovic BV. Neurovascular pathways to neurodegeneration in Alzheimer's disease and other disorders. Nature Reviews. Neuroscience. 2011;**12**:723-738. DOI: 10.1038/nrn3114

[36] Bastías-Candia S, Garrido NA, Zolezzi JM, Inestrosa NC. Recent advances in neuroinflammation therapeutics: PPARs/LXR as neuroinflammatory modulators. Current Pharmaceutical Design. 2016;**22**:1312-1323. DOI: 10.2174/1381612822666151223103038

[37] Ben Halima S, Rajendran L. Membrane anchored and lipid raft targeted β-secretase inhibitors for Alzheimer's disease therapy. Journal of Alzheimer's Disease. 2011;**24**:143-152. DOI: 10.3233/JAD-2011-110269

[38] Larner AJ. Presenilin-1 mutations in Alzheimer's disease: An update on genotype-phenotype relationship. Journal of Alzheimer's Disease. 2013;**37**:653-659. DOI: 10.3233/JAD-130746

[39] Mok KY, Jones EL, Hanney M, Harold D, Sims R, Williams J, et al. Polymorphisms in BACE2 may affect the age of onset Alzheimer's dementia in down syndrome. Neurobiology of Aging. 2013;**35**:1513.e1-1513.e5. DOI: 10.1016/j.neurobiolaging.2013.12.022

[40] Natunen, T, Parrado AR, Helisalmi S, Pursiheimo JP, Sarajärvi T, Mäkinen P, et al. Elucidation of the BACE1 regulating factor GGA3 in Alzheimer's disease. Journal of Alzheimer's Disease. 2013;**37**:217-232. DOI: 10.3233/JAD-130104

[41] Jia SH, Li K, Su W, Li SH, Chen HB. Impairment in the intention formation and execution phases of prospective memory in Parkinson's disease. Frontiers in Neuroscience. 2018;**12**:98. DOI: 10.3389/fnins.2018.00098

[42] Hawkes CH, Del Tredici K, Braak H. A timeline for Parkinson's disease. Parkinsonism & Related Disorders. 2010;**16**:79-84. DOI: 10.1016/j.parkreldis.2009.08.007

[43] Bridi JC, Hirth F. Mechanisms of α-synuclein induced synaptopathy in Parkinson's disease. Frontiers in Neuroscience. 2018;**12**:80. DOI: 10.3389/fnins.2018.00080

[44] Bastías-Candia S, Di Benedetto M, D'Addario C, Candeletti S, Romualdi P. Combined exposure to agriculture pesticides, paraquat and maneb, induces alterations in the N/OFQ-NOPr and PDYN/KOPr systems in rats: Relevance to sporadic Parkinson's disease. Environmental Toxicology. 2015;**30**:656-663. DOI: 10.1002/tox.21943

[45] Murphy DD, Rueter SM, Trojanowski JQ, Lee VM. Synucleins are developmentally expressed, and alpha-synuclein regulates the size of the presynaptic vesicular pool in primary hippocampal neurons. The Journal of Neuroscience. 2000;**20**:3214-3220

[46] Cabin DE, Shimazu K, Murphy D, Cole NB, Gottschalk W, McIlwain KL, et al. Synaptic vesicle depletion correlates with attenuated synaptic responses to prolonged repetitive stimulation in mice lacking alpha-synuclein. The Journal of Neuroscience. 2002;**22**:8797-8807

[47] Larsen KE, Schmitz Y, Troyer MD, Mosharov E, Dietrich P, Quazi AZ, et al. Alpha-synuclein overexpression in PC12 and chromaffin cells impairs catecholamine release by interfering with a late step in exocytosis. The Journal of Neuroscience. 2006;**26**:11915-11922. DOI: 10.1523/JNEUROSCI.3821-06.2006

[48] Burré J, Sharma M, Tsetsenis T, Buchman V, Etherton MR, Südhof TC. Alpha-synuclein promotes SNARE-complex assembly in vivo and in vitro. Science. 2010;**329**:1663-1667. DOI: 10.1126/science.1195227

[49] Lotharius J, Brundin P. Pathogenesis of Parkinson's disease: Dopamine, vesicles and alpha-synuclein. Nature Reviews. Neuroscience. 2002;**3**:932-942. DOI: 10.1038/nrn983

[50] Burré J. The synaptic function of α-synuclein. Journal of Parkinson's Disease. 2015;**5**:699-713. DOI: 10.3233/JPD-150642

[51] Bassil F, Fernagut PO, Bezard E, Pruvost A, Leste-Lasserre T, Hoang QQ, et al. Reducing C-terminal truncation mitigates synucleinopathy and neurodegeneration in a transgenic model of multiple system atrophy. Proceedings of the National Academy of Sciences of the United States of America. 2016;**113**:9593-9598. DOI: 10.1073/pnas.1609291113

[52] Wang W, Nguyen LT, Burlak C, Chegini F, Guo F, Chataway T, et al. Caspase-1 causes truncation and aggregation of the Parkinson's disease-associated protein α-synuclein. Proceedings of the National Academy of Sciences of the United States of America. 2016;**113**:9587-9592. DOI: 10.1073/pnas.1610099113

[53] Li YH, Gao N, Ye YW, Li X, Yu S, Yang H, et al. Alpha-synuclein functions as a negative regulator for expression of tyrosine hydroxylase. Acta Neurologica Belgica. 2011;111: 130-135

[54] Butler B, Goodwin S, Saha K, Becker J, Sambo D, Davari P, et al. Dopamine transporter activity is modulated by alpha-synuclein. The Journal of Biological Chemistry. 2015;290:29542-29554. DOI: 10.1074/jbc.M115.691592

[55] Heneka MT, Golenbock DT, Latz E. Innate immunity in Alzheimer's disease. Nature Immunology. 2015;16:229-236. DOI: 10.1038/ni.3102

[56] Heneka MT, Carson MJ, El Khoury J, Landreth GE, Brosseron F, Feinstein DL, et al. Neuroinflammation in Alzheimer's disease. Lancet Neurology. 2015;14:388-405. DOI: 10.1016/S1474-4422(15)70016-5

[57] Malipiero U, Koedel U, Pfister HW, Levéen P, Bürki K, Reith W, et al. TGFbeta receptor II gene deletion in leucocytes prevents cerebral vasculitis in bacterial meningitis. Brain. 2006;129:2404-2415. DOI: 10.1093/brain/awl192

[58] Strle K, Zhou JH, Shen WH, Broussard SR, Johnson RW, Freund GG, et al. Interleukin-10 in the brain. Critical Reviews in Immunology. 2001;21:427-449. DOI: 10.1615/CritRev Immunol.v21.i5.20

[59] Landreth G, Reed-Geaghan E. Toll-like receptors in Alzheimer's disease. Current Topics in Microbiology and Immunology. 2009;336:137-153. DOI: 10.1007/978-3-642-00549-7_8

[60] Hanke M, Kielian T. Toll-like receptors in health and disease in the brain: Mechanisms and therapeutic potential. Clinical Science (London). 2011;121:367-387. DOI: 10.1042/ CS20110164

[61] Mishra BB, Mishra PK, Teale JM. Expression and distribution of toll-like receptors in the brain during murine neurocysticercosis. Journal of Neuroimmunology. 2006;181:46-56. DOI: 10.1016/j.jneuroim.2006.07.019

[62] Atmaca HT, Kul O, Karakus E, Terzi OS, Canpolat S, Anteplioglu T. Astrocytes, microglia/macrophages, and neurons expressing toll-like receptor 11 contribute to innate immunity against encephalitic toxoplasma gondii infection. Neuroscience. 2014;269:184-191. DOI: 10.1016/j.neuroscience.2014.03.049

[63] Doorn KJ, Lucassen PJ, Boddeke HW, Prins M, Berendse HW, Drukarch B, et al. Emerging roles of microglial activation and non-motor symptoms in Parkinson's disease. Progress in Neurobiology. 2012;98:222-238. DOI: 10.1016/j.pneurobio.2012.06.005

[64] Blandini F. Neural and immune mechanisms in the pathogenesis of Parkinson's disease. Journal of Neuroimmune Pharmacology. 2013;8:189-201. DOI: 10.1007/s11481-013-9435-y

[65] Andreasson KI, Bachstetter AD, Colonna M, Ginhoux F, Holmes C, Lamb B, et al. Targetin innate immunity for neurodegenerative disorders of the central nervous system. Journal of Neurochemistry. 2016;138:653-693. DOI: 10.1111/jnc.13667

[66] Reed-Geaghan EG, Savage JC, Hise AG, Landreth GE. CD14 and toll-like receptors 2 and 4 are required for fibrillar ab-stimulated microglial activation. The Journal of Neuroscience. 2009;29:11982-11992. DOI: 10.1523/JNEUROSCI.3158-09.2009

[67] Dursun E, Gezen-Ak D, Hanağası H, Bilgiç B, Lohmann E, Ertan S, et al. The interleukin 1 alpha, interleukin 1 beta, interleukin 6 and alpha-2-macroglobulin serum levels in patients with early or late onset Alzheimer's disease, mild cognitive impairment or Parkinson's disease. Journal of Neuroimmunology. 2015;283:50-57. DOI: 10.1016/j.jneuroim.2015.04.014

[68] Cameron B, Landreth GE. Inflammation, microglia, and Alzheimer's disease. Neurobiology of Disease. 2010;37:503-509. DOI: 10.1016/j.nbd.2009.10.006

[69] Wake H, Moorhouse AJ, Miyamoto A, Nabekura J. Microglia: Actively surveying and shaping neuronal circuit structure and function. Trends in Neurosciences. 2013;36:209-217. DOI: 10.1016/j.tins.2012.11.007

[70] Crehan J, Hardy J, Pocock J. Blockage of CR1 prevents activation of rodent microglia. Neurobiology of Disease. 2013;54:139-149. DOI: 10.1016/j.nbd.2013.02.003

[71] Griciuc A, Serrano-Pozo A, Parrado AR, Lesinski AN, Asselin CN, Mullin K, et al. Alzheimer's disease risk gene CD33 inhibits microglial uptake of amyloid beta. Neuron. 2013;78:631-643. DOI: 10.1016/j.neuron.2013.04.014

[72] Wang Y, Cella M, Mallinson KJ, Ulrich JD, Young KL, Robinette ML, et al. TREM2 lipid sensing sustains the microglial response in an Alzheimer's disease model. Cell. 2015;160:1061-1071. DOI: 10.1016/j.cell.2015.01.049

[73] Zhao Y, Wu X, Li X, Jiang LL, Gui X, Liu Y, et al. TREM2 is a receptor for β-amyloid that mediates microglial function. Neuron. 2018;97:1023-1031.e7. DOI: 10.1016/j.neuron.2018.01.031

[74] Guerreiro R, Wojtas A, Bras J, Carrasquillo M, Rogaeva E, Majounie E, et al. TREM2 variants in Alzheimer's disease. The New England Journal of Medicine. 2013;368:117-127. DOI: 10.1056/NEJMoa1211851

[75] Brosseron F, Traschütz A, Widmann CN, Kummer MP, Tacik P, Santarelli F, et al. Characterization and clinical use of inflammatory cerebrospinal fluid protein markers in Alzheimer's disease. Alzheimer's Research & Therapy. 2018;10:25. DOI: 10.1186/s13195-018-0353-3

[76] Leyns CEG, Ulrich JD, Finn MB, Stewart FR, Koscal LJ, Remolina Serrano J, et al. TREM2 deficiency attenuates neuroinflammation and protects against neurodegeneration in a mouse model of tauopathy. Proceedings of the National Academy of Sciences of the United States of America. 2017;114:11524-11529. DOI: 10.1073/pnas.1710311114

[77] Bemiller SM, McCray TJ, Allan K, Formica SV, Xu G, Wilson G, et al. TREM2 deficiency exacerbates tau pathology through dysregulated kinase signaling in a mouse model of tauopathy. Molecular Neurodegeneration. 2017 Oct 16;12:74. DOI: 10.1186/s13024-017-0216-6

[78] Stefanova N, Fellner L, Reindl M, Masliah E, Poewe W, Wenning GK. Toll-like receptor 4 promotes α-synuclein clearance and survival of nigral dopaminergic neurons. The American Journal of Pathology. 2011;179:954-963. DOI: 10.1016/j.ajpath.2011.04.013

[79] Fellner L, Irschick R, Schanda K, Reindl M, Klimaschewski L, Poewe W, et al. Toll-like receptor 4 is required for α-synuclein dependent activation of microglia and astroglia. Glia. 2013;**61**:349-360. DOI: 10.1002/glia.22437

[80] Kim C, Ho DH, Suk JE, You S, Michael S, Kang J, et al. Neuron-released oligomeric α-synuclein is an endogenous agonist of TLR2 for paracrine activation of microglia. Nature Communications. 2013;**4**:1562. DOI: 10.1038/ncomms2534

[81] Sanchez-Guajardo V, Tentillier N, Romero-Ramos M. The relation between α-synuclein and microglia in Parkinson's disease: Recent developments. Neuroscience. 2015;**302**:47-58. DOI: 10.1016/j.neuroscience.2015.02.008

[82] Ganguly U, Chakrabarti SS, Kaur U, Mukherjee A, Chakrabarti S. Alpha-synuclein, proteotoxicity and Parkinson's disease: Search for neuroprotective therapy. Current Neuropharmacology. 2017;**15**. DOI: 10.2174/1570159X15666171129100944

[83] Lee HJ, Suk JE, Patrick C, Bae EJ, Cho JH, Rho S, et al. Direct transfer of alpha-synuclein from neuron to astroglia causes inflammatory responses in synucleinopathies. The Journal of Biological Chemistry. 2010;**285**:9262-9272. DOI: 10.1074/jbc.M109.081125

[84] Farina C, Aloisi F, Meinl E. Astrocytes are active players in cerebral innate immunity. Trends in Immunology. 2007;**28**:138-145. DOI: 10.1016/j.it.2007.01.005

[85] Ambrosini E, Aloisi F. Chemokines and glial cells: A complex network in the central nervous system. Neurochemical Research. 2004;**29**:1017-1038. DOI: 10.1023/B:N ERE.0000021246.96864.89

[86] Morales I, Rodriguez M. Self-induced accumulation of glutamate in striatal astrocytes and basal ganglia excitotoxicity. Glia. 2012;**60**:1481-1494. DOI: 10.1002/glia.22368

[87] Roodveldt C, Labrador-Garrido A, Gonzalez-Rey E, Lachaud CC, Guilliams T, Fernandez-Montesinos R, et al. Preconditioning of microglia by α-synuclein strongly affects the response induced by toll-like receptor (TLR) stimulation. PLoS One. 2013;**8**:e79160. DOI: 10.1371/journal.pone.0079160

[88] Aktas O, Ullrich O, Infante-Duarte C, Nitsch R, Zipp F. Neuronal damage in brain inflammation. Archives of Neurology. 2007;**64**:185-189. DOI: 10.1001/archneur.64.2.185

[89] Little AR, Benkovic SA, Miller DB, O'Callaghan JP. Chemically induced neuronal damage and gliosis: Enhanced expression of the proinflammatory chemokine, monocyte chemoattractant protein (MCP)-1, without a corresponding increase in proinflammatory cytokines. Neuroscience. 2002;**115**:307-320. DOI: 10.1016/S0306-4522(02)00359-7

[90] Patel NS, Paris D, Mathura V, Quadros AN, Crawford FC, Mullan MJ. Inflammatory cytokine levels correlate with amyloid load in transgenic mouse models of Alzheimer's disease. Journal of Neuroinflammation. 2005;**2**:9. DOI: 10.1186/1742-2094-2-9

[91] Cai Q, Tammineni P. Mitochondrial aspects of synaptic dysfunction in Alzheimer's disease. Journal of Alzheimer's Disease. DOI: 10.3233/JAD-160726

[92] Kerr JS, Adriaanse BA, Greig NH, Mattson MP, Cader MZ, Bohr VA, et al. Mitophagy and Alzheimer's disease: Cellular and molecular mechanisms. Trends in Neurosciences. 2017;**40**:151-166. DOI: 10.1016/j.tins.2017.01.002

[93] Zolezzi JM, Silva-Alvarez C, Ordenes D, Godoy JA, Carvajal FJ, Santos MJ, et al. Peroxisome proliferator-activated receptor (PPAR) γ and PPARα agonists modulate mitochondrial fusion-fission dynamics: Relevance to reactive oxygen species (ROS)-related neurodegenerative disorders? PLoS One. 2013;**8**:e64019. DOI: 10.1371/journal.pone.0064019

[94] Ordonez DG, Lee MK, Feany MB. α-Synuclein induces mitochondrial dysfunction through spectrin and the actin cytoskeleton. Neuron. 2018;**97**:108-124.e6. DOI: 10.1016/j.neuron.2017.11.036

[95] Chen H, Zhang SM, Hern'an MA, et al. Nonsteroidal anti-inflammatory drugs and the risk of Parkinson disease. Archives of Neurology. 2003;**60**:1059-1064

[96] Vlad SC, Miller DR, Kowall NW, Felson DT. Protective effects of NSAIDs on the development of Alzheimer disease. Neurology. 2008;**70**:1672-1677

[97] Pimplikar SW. Neuroinflammation in Alzheimer's disease: From pathogenesis to a therapeutic target. Journal of Clinical Immunology. 2014;**34**:S64-S69. DOI: 10.1007/s10875-014-0032-5

[98] Farr JN, Roforth MM, Fujita K, Nicks KM, Cunningham JM, Atkinson EJ, et al. Effects of age and estrogen on skeletal gene expression in humans as assessed by RNA sequencing. PLoS One. 2015;**10**:e0138347. DOI: 10.1371/journal.pone.0138347

[99] García-Velázquez L, Arias C. The emerging role of Wnt signaling dysregulation in the understanding and modification of age-associated diseases. Ageing Research Reviews. 2017;**37**:135-145. DOI: 10.1016/j.arr.2017.06.001

[100] Lambert C, Cisternas P, Inestrosa NC. Role of Wnt signaling in central nervous system injury. Molecular Neurobiology. 2016;**53**:2297-2311. DOI: 10.1007/s12035-015-9138-x

[101] Godoy JA, Rios JA, Zolezzi JM, Braidy N, Inestrosa NC. Signaling pathway cross talk in Alzheimer's disease. Cell Communication and Signaling: CCS. 2014;**12**:23. DOI: 10.1186/1478-811X-12-23

[102] Tapia-Rojas C, Inestrosa NC. Wnt signaling loss accelerates the appearance of neuropathological hallmarks of Alzheimer's disease in J20-APP transgenic and wild-type mice. Journal of Neurochemistry. 2018;**144**:443-465. DOI: 10.1111/jnc.14278

[103] Cisternas P, Salazar P, Silva-Álvarez C, Barros LF, Inestrosa NC. Activation of Wnt signaling in cortical neurons enhances glucose utilization through glycolysis. The Journal of Biological Chemistry. 2016;**291**:25950-25964. DOI: 10.1074/jbc.M116.735373

[104] Berwick DC, Harvey K. LRRK2 functions as a Wnt signaling scaffold, bridging cytosolic proteins and membrane-localized LRP6. Human Molecular Genetics. 2012;**21**:4966-4979. DOI: 10.1093/hmg/dds342

[105] Rawal N, Corti O, Sacchetti P, Ardilla-Osorio H, Sehat B, Brice A, et al. Parkin protects dopaminergic neurons from excessive Wnt/beta-catenin signaling. Biochemical and Bio-physical Research Communications. 2009;**388**:473-478. DOI: 10. 1016/j.bbrc.2009.07.014

[106] Arenas E. Wnt signaling in midbrain dopaminergic neuron development and regenera-tive medicine for Parkinson's disease. Journal of Molecular Cell Biology. 2014;**6**:42-53. DOI: 10.1093/jmcb/mju001

[107] Yi H, Patel AK, Sodhi CP, Hackam DJ, Hackam AS. Novel role for the innate immune receptor toll-like receptor 4 (TLR4) in the regulation of the Wnt signaling pathway and photoreceptor apoptosis. PLoS One. 2012;**7**:e36560. DOI: 10.1371/journal.pone.0036560

[108] Trinath J, Holla S, Mahadik K, Prakhar P, Singh V, Balaji KN. The WNT signaling path-way contributes to dectin-1-dependent inhibition of toll-like receptor-induced inflam-matory signature. Molecular and Cellular Biology. 2014;**34**:4301-4314. DOI: 10.1128/MCB.00641-14

[109] Ishitani T. Context-dependent dual and opposite roles of nemo-like kinase in the Wnt/β-catenin signaling. Cell Cycle. 2012;**11**:1743-1745. DOI: 10.4161/cc.20183

[110] Ishitani T, Kishida S, Hyodo-Miura J, Ueno N, Yasuda J, Waterman M, et al. The TAK1-NLK mitogen-activated protein kinase cascade functions in the Wnt-5a/Ca(2+) pathway to antagonize Wnt/beta-catenin signaling. Molecular and Cellular Biology. 2003;**23**:131-139. DOI: 10.1128/MCB.23.1.131-139.2003

[111] Xie X, Zhang D, Zhao B, Lu MK, You M, Condorelli G, et al. IkappaB kinase epsilon and TANK-binding kinase 1 activate AKT by direct phosphorylation. Proceedings of the National Academy of Sciences of the United States of America. 2011;**108**:6474-6479. DOI: 10.1073/pnas.1016132108

[112] Li N, Zhang X, Dong H, Zhang S, Sun J, Qian Y. Lithium ameliorates LPS-induced astrocytes activation partly via inhibition of toll-like receptor 4 expression. Cellular Physiology and Biochemistry. 2016;**38**:714-725. DOI: 10.1159/000443028

Neurodegenerative Diseases Associated with Mutations in *SLC25A46*

Zhuo Li, Jesse Slone, Lingqian Wu and
Taosheng Huang

Additional information is available at the end of the chapter

http://dx.doi.org/10.5772/intechopen.79992

Abstract

Neurodegenerative diseases present substantial clinical challenges. Their processes have been linked with various genetic causes, including mutations of genes encoding proteins associated with mitochondrial dynamics. Biallelic mutations in *SLC25A46* have been identified as novel causes of a wide spectrum of neurological diseases with recessive inheritance, including optic atrophy, Charcot-Marie-Tooth neuropathy (CMT) type 2A neuropathy, Leigh syndrome, progressive myoclonic ataxia, and lethal congenital pontocerebellar hypoplasia. SLC25A46 (solute carrier family 25 member 46) is a membrane transit protein that is expressed in the mitochondrial outer membrane where it plays a major role in mitochondrial dynamics and cristae maintenance. This chapter presents recent findings on: (1) the clinical heterogeneity of SLC25A46-related neuropathies; (2) the *SLC25A46* mutation spectrum and associated genotype-phenotype correlation; and (3) pathophysiological functions of SLC25A46 as characterized in cells and mouse models. A better understanding of the etiology of *SLC25146*-linked diseases will elucidate therapeutic perspectives.

Keywords: neurodegeneration, SLC25A46, mitochondrial dynamics, optic atrophy, CMT-2 neuropathy, pontocerebellar hypoplasia

1. Introduction

Mitochondria have long been recognized as critical organelles for cellular energy generation. They produce ~90% of neuronal adenosine triphosphate (ATP), which is continuously required for maintaining the complex morphology and specialized functions of neurons, including electrical excitability and synaptic transmission [1], and are regenerated continuously in postmitotic neurons through biogenesis. In addition to undergoing the dynamic processes of mitochondrial fission and fusion, mitochondria are transported bidirectionally within neurites, in which they are distributed purposefully, facilitating energy transmission over long distances to meet local demands and, when necessary, undergo controlled degradation by mitophagy [2, 3]. Thus, mitochondrial dynamics play critical roles in neuronal homeostasis and survival.

Recent evidence suggests that abnormal mitochondrial dynamics may contribute to both familial and sporadic neurodegenerative diseases [4]. Most proteins related to mitochondrial dynamics are encoded by genes in the nucleus. Mutations in such nuclear-encoded genes can cause monogenic disorders in which mitochondrial dysfunction is unequivocally central to the pathogenesis of the disease. For example, mutations in *MFN1/2* and *OPA1* cause Charcot-Marie-Tooth neuropathy (CMT) type 2A [5–7] and autosomal dominant optic atrophy (ADOA) [8–10], respectively. A dominant negative allele of *DRP1* was identified in a neonate with a lethal mitochondrial and peroxisomal fission defect associated with abnormal brain development, optic atrophy, and various other congenital anomalies [11]. Defects in proteins involved in axonal transport have also been identified in patients with CMT and related neuropathies [12–14]. In addition, there is increasing evidence linking mitochondrial dysfunction to neuronal loss in age-related neurodegenerative disorders, including Alzheimer's disease and Parkinson's disease [15, 16].

Recent studies have implicated the 46th isoform of subfamily A of the solute carrier (SLC) family 25, termed SLC25A46, in mitochondrial dysfunction pathology. SLC25A46 is a mitochondrial outer membrane protein that was shown recently to be involved in mitochondrial dynamics, either playing a role in mitochondrial fission or serving as a regulator of mitofusin (MFN)1/2 oligomerization [17, 18]. Disorders caused by recessive *SLC25A46* mutations were defined recently as a new syndrome (introduced and elaborated in Section 3.1) that has a broad clinical spectrum of neurological phenotypes, including peripheral neuropathy, early-onset optic atrophy, cerebellar degeneration, and congenital pontocerebellar hypoplasia (PCH), with variable ages of onset and severities [17, 19–26]. In this chapter, we will focus on the phenotypic and genetic characteristics of *SLC25A46*-related neurological diseases and our current understanding of the pathophysiological mechanisms linking dysfunctional SLC25A46 to neurodegeneration.

2. SLC25 family and the discovery of *SLC25A46*

SLC25A46 belongs to the solute carrier family 25 (SLC25), a superfamily that contains 53 nuclear-encoded mitochondrial carrier proteins in humans [27]. SLC25 members are characterized by the presence of three tandem repeats of about 100 amino acids, each containing two transmembrane alpha helices linked by a large loop [28]. The mature carrier protein thus consists of six transmembrane helices that form an aqueous pore and have a highly conserved consensus sequence, P-X-[D/E]-X-X-[R/K], at the C-terminal ends of the three odd-numbered transmembrane alpha helices, whose charged residues form salt bridges that close the pore on the matrix side [29]. SLC25 proteins may shuttle a variety of solutes across the mitochondrial membrane to participate in various metabolic pathways [30]. Although common mechanisms of substrate translocation have been proposed, SLC25 members vary greatly in their size, the nature of substrates they transport, the modes of transport employed, and the driving forces they employ [30–32].

A number of genetic conditions associated with SLC25 mitochondrial transporters have been characterized biochemically and genetically [33]. SLC25 members mediate a variety of cellular functions, and mutations in SLC25 genes have been linked to various defects, such as carnitine/acylcarnitine carrier deficiency (OMIM 212138), HHH syndrome (OMIM 238970), aspartate/glutamate isoform 1 and 2 deficiencies (OMIM 612949, 603471, 605814), congenital Amish

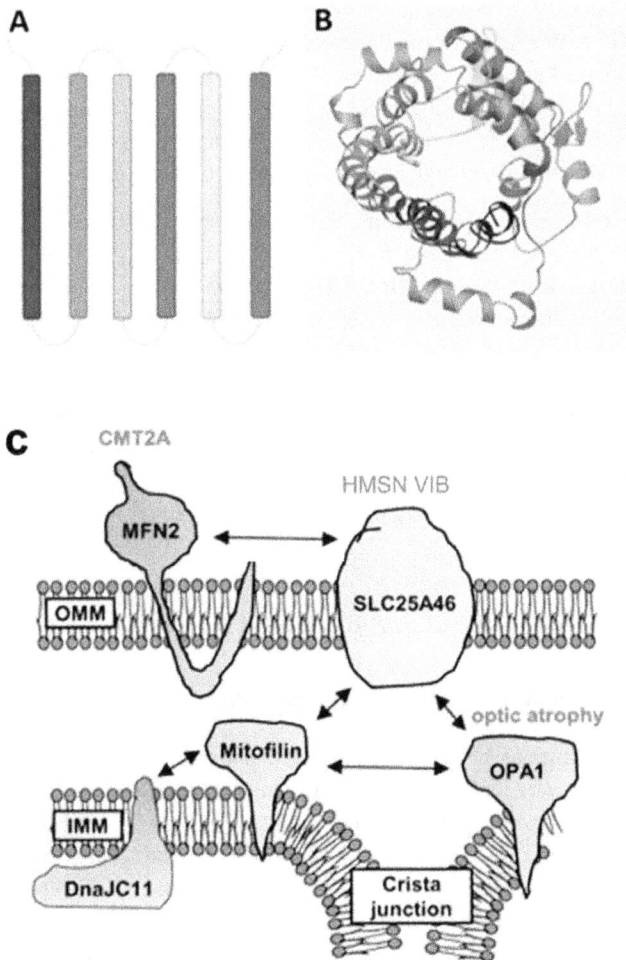

Figure 1. Schematic diagram of SLC25A46 structure and its interactions. (A) SLC25A46 consists of six conserved transmembrane alpha helices. (B) 3D structure of SLC25A46. (C) Potential interactions of SLC25A46 with dynamic proteins.

microcephaly (OMIM 607196), neuropathy with bilateral striatal necrosis (OMIM 613710), congenital sideroblastic anemia (OMIM 205950), neonatal epileptic encephalopathy (OMIM 609304), and citrate carrier deficiency (OMIM 190315) [33]. These disorders are characterized by specific metabolic dysfunctions related to the role of the particular carrier that has been affected. Most disease-related SLC25 members have been characterized in terms of substrate identification and associated metabolic pathways, with the exception of two orphan SLC25 members, namely SLC25A38 and SLC25A46 [33].

SLC25A46 was first mapped to chromosome 5 by genomic sequence analysis in 2006 [27]. Its location was further refined to chromosome 5q22.1 based on sequence alignment with NCBI's standard reference human assembly sequence, that is, the Genome Reference Consortium Human genome build 38. The largest transcript isoform of *SLC25A46* contains eight exons, which encode a 418-amino acid protein. Quantitative real-time polymerase chain reaction (PCR) experiments in rodents have demonstrated variable expression of *SLC25A46* in all tissues examined, with the highest levels occurring in the hindbrain, spinal cord, and coronal brain sections containing the corpus callosum, fornix, optic chiasm, thalamus, hypothalamus, midbrain, pons, and cerebellum, with particularly high levels in mouse embryo cerebellum [27].

Given the typical SLC25 molecular structure, the primary sequence of the SLC25A46 protein has been predicted to form six conserved transmembrane alpha helices, TM1–TM6, spanning a region between amino acids 100–418 (**Figure 1**) [22]. However, the otherwise highly conserved P-X-(D/E)-X-X-(R/K) consensus sequence characteristic of SLC25 proteins is altered in SLC25A46. Moreover, the N-terminus of SLC25A46 is about five times longer than that of other members of the family (~100 vs. <20 amino acids). These unusual characteristics suggest that SLC25A46 is unlikely to have a conventional metabolite carrier function. Recently, studies have proposed that unlike most SLC25 members that are located in the inner mitochondrial membrane, SLC25A46 may be anchored to the outer mitochondrial membrane where it may act as a regulator of mitochondrial dynamics rather than as a substrate transporter.

3. Clinical phenotypes of *SLC25A46*-related diseases

3.1. Hereditary motor and sensory neuropathy type VIB (HMSN6B)

In 2015, recessive mutations in *SLC25A46* in eight patients from four unrelated families of various ethnic origins were first reported. The proband phenotypes encompassed ADOA-like optic atrophy, CMT-like axonal peripheral neuropathy, and cerebellar atrophy with a variable age of onset and disease course (**Table 1**) [17]. This new neurodegenerative syndrome is now defined as HMSN6B in OMIM (OMIM: 616505). ADOA and CMT type 2 are hereditary neurodegenerative disorders commonly caused by mutations in the mitochondrial fusion genes *OPA1* and *MFN2*, respectively. However, both diseases lack a genetic diagnosis in up to 60% of patients due to genetic heterogeneity [34, 35].

SLC25A46 provides a new locus in genetic testing for patients with ADOA and CMT-like phenotypes. Indeed, four independent clinical reports published in 2016 and 2017 identified

ID	SLC25A46 mutations	SLC25A46 proteins	Age of onset	Age of death	Optic atrophy	Peripheral neuropathy	Cerebellar or brainstem atrophy	Hypotonia or myopathy	Ataxia	Lactate	Other features	Mitochondrial dynamics
UK family Abrams et al. [17]	c.165_166insC; c.746G>A	p.His56fs*94; p.Gly249Asp	5 y/8 y	Alive (40 y/43 y)	+	+	−	−	−	Normal	Normal CSF examination, oxidative enzyme activity, no ragged red fibers.	n.k.
PL family Abrams et al. [17]	c.1005A>T	p.Glu335Asp	1 y/2 y	Alive (13 mo/11.5 y)	+	+	+	+	+	↑	Developmental delay, 3-MG ↑ in urine.	Increased mitochondria.
IT family Abrams et al. [17]	c.1018C>T	p.Arg340Cys	2 y	Alive (51 y)	+	+	+	+	+	↑	CK ↑(225, NR<170 U/L), lactic acid at upper end of normal range.	Hyperfilamentous.
US family Abrams et al. [17]	c.882_885dupTTAC; c.998C>T	p.Asn296fs*297; p.Pro333Leu	Prenatal	105 d	+	+	+	+	n.k.	n.k.	Facial and hand dysmorphism, meconium aspiration.	n.k.
Moroccan family Nguyen et al. [21]	c.283+3G>T	p.?	Prenatal	7 d	+	n.k.	+	+	n.k.	↑	Club foot posture, lactate-to-pyruvate ratio ↑ and all individual complexes ↓ in fibroblasts.	Mitochondrial fragmentation.
Pakistani origin family Charlesworth et al. [19]	c.413T>G	p.Leu138Arg	n.k.	Alive (15 y/20 y)	+	+	+	+	+	n.k.	Comprised exotropia, difficulty initiating saccades, spasticity, scoliosis. Old brother with mild phenotypes.	n.k.
Saudi family Sulaiman et al. [26]	c.775C>T	p.Arg259Cys	28 y	Alive	+	−	−	+	n.k.	Normal	No ragged red fiber or cytochrome c deficiency, intact sensation and coordination, unremarkable acylcarnitine profile, amino acids, CK and urine organic acids.	Occasional enlarged mitochondria.
Tunisian family Hammer et al. [23]	c.1018C>T	p.Arg340Cys	1 y/6 y	Alive (22 y/19 y)	+	+	±	n.k.	+	n.k.	Dysarthria, gait instability, Babinski sign, abolished Achilles reflexes, finger-nose dysmetria, severe sensorimotor demyelination.	n.k.

ID	SLC25A46 mutations	SLC25A46 proteins	Age of onset	Age of death	Optic atrophy	Peripheral neuropathy	Cerebellar or brainstem atrophy	Hypotonia or myopathy	Ataxia	Lactate	Other features	Mitochondrial dynamics
Algerian family 1 Hammer et al. [23]	c.1018C>T	p.Arg340Cys	2 y	Alive (31 y)	+	+	±	n.k.	+	n.k.	Subtle white matter changes in cerebellum, increased tendon reflexes, no Achilles reflex, positive Hoffmann sign, no Babinski sign.	n.k.
Algerian family 2 Hammer et al. [23]	c.479G>C	p.Trp160Ser	23 y	Alive (26 y)	–	n.k.	n.k.	n.k.	+	n.k.	Abolished vibration sense, at ankles, nystagmus and saccadic pursuit, scoliosis.	n.k.
Family 1 Wan et al. [22]	c.1022T>C	p.Leu341Pro	Prenatal	14 d/28 d	n.k.	n.k.	+	+	n.k.	Normal	PCH, severe global developmental delay, normal respiratory chain enzymes in muscle and liver.	Increase in mitochondrial length.
Family 2 Wan et al. [22]	g.chr5:110738771_110746700del	p.?	Prenatal	42 d	+	+	+	+	n.k.	↑	PCH, occasional myoclonic jerks; EEG: generalized slowing with abnormal theta rhythm, no epileptic discharges, sibling with same phenotype.	n.k.
Dutch family Dijk et al. [25]	c.691C>T g.chr5:110742638_110745029del	p.Arg231*; p.?	Prenatal	1 d	+	n.k.	+	+	n.k.	n.k.	PCH, all three children died within 1 day after birth, lack of spontaneous respiration, profound muscle weakness. Convulsion, spinal motor neuron degeneration.	n.k.
German family Braunisch et al. [24]	c.736A>T	p. Arg 246 *	Prenatal	1 d/23 d	n.k.	n.k.	+	+	n.k.	↑	PCH, seizures, EEG: low amplitudes with sharp waves, epileptiform discharges without clinical equivalents, thrombocytes ↑, lung hypoplasia,	n.k.

ID	SLC25A46 mutations	SLC25A46 proteins	Age of onset	Age of death	Optic atrophy	Peripheral neuropathy	Cerebellar or brainstem atrophy	Hypotonia or myopathy	Ataxia	Lactate	Other features	Mitochondrial dynamics
Italian family Braunisch et al. [24]	c.42C>G; c.462+1G>A	p.Tyr14 *; P. ?	Prenatal	1 d/18 d	n.k.	n.k.	+	+	n.k.	n.k.	bradycardia at birth, green amniotic fluid. PCH, floppy infant, little respiratory effort and voluntary movements; EMG: neurogenic lesion; loss of spinal motor neurons, normal CK levels, serum transferrin IEF, two siblings were hypotonic and died immediately after birth.	n.k.
French Canadian family Janer et al. [20]	c.425C>T	p.Thr142Ile; (instable protein)	Birth	15 mo	+	n.k.	+	+	n.k.	↑	Leigh syndrome, psychomotor delay, growth retardation, mild spastic diplegia; motor delay; fever, convulsion, gasping respirations, bilateral intranuclear ophthalmoplegia, hyperreflexia, mild spasticity.	Mitochondrial hyperfusion in fibroblast.

Note: y, year; mo, month; d, day; n.k., not known; ↑, increase.

Table 1. Clinical phenotypes associated with SLC25A46 mutations.

homogenous *SLC25A46* mutations in an additional nine patients (age range, 7 days to 28 years) from five unrelated families who presented with neurological phenotypes similar to the core features of HMSN6B. Among these nine patients, eight had optic atrophy (the exception was a patient with an age of onset 23 years) and eight had cerebellar atrophy (the exception was a 28-year-old patient without remarkable cerebellar atrophy or axonal neuropathy) (**Table 1**) [19, 21, 23, 26]. Beyond the key clinical features of optic atrophy, peripheral neuropathy, and cerebellar atrophy, the presently documented population of 17 patients with HMSN6B (or an HMSN6B-like condition) exhibited other clinical symptoms sporadically, including ataxia, hypotonia, myoclonus, dysmetria, nystagmus, speech difficulties, abnormal brain imaging, and elevated lactic acid (**Table 1**). The clinical manifestations, medical examination findings, and differential diagnoses for these patients were strongly suggestive of a progressive mitochondrial disorder.

3.2. *SLC25A46*-related PCH and Leigh syndrome

A recent study reported the identification of *SLC25A46* loss-of-function mutations in four patients from two unrelated families with a diagnosis of severe congenital PCH, leading to very early mortality [22]. Then, two independent groups reported an additional seven patients from three unrelated families with severe PCH associated with truncating mutations of *SLC25A46* (**Table 1**) [24, 25].

PCH is a rare, heterogeneous group of prenatal onset neurodegenerative disorders, mainly (but not exclusively) affecting the cerebellum and pons. The current PCH classification scheme includes 10 distinct PCH subtypes defined by clinical features and genetic etiology. PCH1 is distinguished from the other PCH subtypes by its association with spinal muscular atrophy due to spinal motoneuron degeneration; it often leads to early death. All patients with obvious loss-of-function *SLC25A46* genotypes in the literature suffered severe lethal congenital PCH, presenting with the phenotypic hallmarks of cerebellar and brainstem degeneration as well as spinal muscular atrophy, respiratory failure, early death, occasional optic nerve atrophy, and axonal neuropathy. Based on these features, SLC25A46-associated PCH could be classified as PCH1, and perhaps a new PCH1 subtype, PCH1D, clinically distinguished from other PCH1 subtypes (mutations in *VRK1*, *EXOSC3*, and *EXOSC8* are associated with PCH1A, PCH1B, and PCH1C, respectively) [25]. However, the most severe clinical presentation associated with *SLC25A46* mutations is probably not restricted to PCH. A homozygous *SLC25A46* mutation that resulted in the complete absence of the protein was identified recently in a terminally ill child with progressive brain lesions consistent with those seen in Leigh syndrome (**Table 1**) [20].

Cerebellar and brainstem atrophy are shared phenotypic features of PCH, Leigh syndrome, and most variant *SLC25A46*-related HMSN6B cases. Meanwhile, optic nerve and peripheral nerve axonal pathology are seen consistently in HMSN6B. Features that are prominent in later-onset cases might be overlooked or not assessed in neonatally lethal cases. Thus, *SLC25A46*-related PCH or Leigh syndrome could be extreme forms of HMSN6B.

To sum up, *SLC25A46*-related neurological disease has high clinical heterogeneity. Patients with biallelic *SLC25A46* mutations show high phenotypic variability with respect to age of onset, clinical features, and disease course. The severity of presentation even varies between siblings. The phenotype spectrum ranges from severe disease at birth with early death to manifestation in late childhood with survival beyond 50 years of age.

4. Mutation spectrum of *SLC25A46* and genotype-phenotype correlation

4.1. Mutation spectrum of *SLC25A46*

The *SLC25A46* gene, located on chromosome 5q22.1, spans approximately 27 kb and is composed of eight exons. The main protein isoform has 418 amino acids and is encoded by a 1257-nucleotide-long open reading frame. Since *SLC25A46* mutations associated with neurological disease were first reported in 2015, more than 28 patients with various mutations from 16 unrelated families have been diagnosed genetically, most by whole-exome sequencing, leading to the discovery of a total of 18 pathogenic mutations in the last 2 years (**Figure 2**). Of these, 50% are missense mutations; 16.7% are nonsense mutations; 11.1% are splice variants; and 22.2% are micro-deletions, insertions, or duplications. The mutation sizes range from a single nucleotide polymorphism to a 2.4-kb deletion. Although some mutations have been found in all exons except exons 2, 6, and 7, 50% of the mutations are located in exon 8, the largest exon, which accounts for half of the *SLC25A46* open reading frame (**Figure 2**). Although there is no suspected mutation hotspot site, the c.1081C>T variant was observed in 3 of 16 independent families (**Table 1**). The identification and genetic diagnosis of additional cases in the future may reveal a *SLC25A46* mutation pattern.

4.2. Genotype-phenotype correlation

A systemic genotype-phenotype analysis of all available cases indicates that phenotype severity correlates strongly with the magnitude of SLC25A46 protein level reduction caused by each

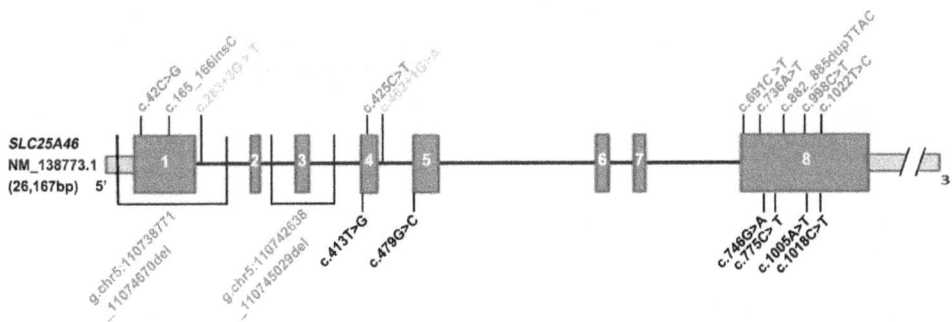

Figure 2. Schematic diagram of reported pathogenic SLC25A46 variants. Exons 1–8 are represented by blue blocks. Mutations are color coded as follows: red, nonsense and missense mutations that would be expected to destabilize the protein; blue, micro-deletions/insertions/duplications; orange, splice-site mutations; and black, regular missense mutations.

mutation. As shown in **Table 1**, very severe *SLC25A46*-related disease has been linked to mutations that yield markedly reduced SLC25A46 levels, including homozygous or compound heterozygous nonsense mutations, (c.691C>T, p.Arg231*; c.736A>T, p.Arg246*; c.42C>G, p.Tyr14*), a splice site variant (c.462+1G>A), and a micro-deletion (g.chr5: 110738771_11074670del). In addition, Wan et al. and Janer et al. verified that the three missense mutations c.1022T>C (p.Leu341Pro), c.998C>T (p.Pro333Leu), and c.425C>T (p. Thr142Ile) destabilize the protein without nonsense-mediated mRNA decay, causing a marked loss of SLC25A46 function. Such protein-depriving mutations lead to severe clinical symptoms of PCH or Leigh syndrome. In contrast, missense mutations of *SLC25A46* that are associated with normal or mildly reduced protein levels tend to result in a relatively mild phenotype. For instance, stable expression of the p.Gly249Asp mutant protein produces low-severity manifestations of optic atrophy spectrum disorder [17, 22] (**Table 1**). Thus, the more stable, functional, and abundant the mutant protein, the less severe the clinical manifestations.

In conclusion, the main molecular causes of *SLC25A46*-related neurological disease appear to be SLC25A46 loss of function or deficiency. The recessive inheritance pattern observed in all pathogenic *SLC25A46* mutation-affected individuals and families thus far contrast with the dominant inheritance pattern observed with other mitochondrial dynamic genes, including *OPA1*, *MFN1/2*, and *DRP1*, for which haplo-insufficiency and dominant negative effects are observed [8, 36, 37].

5. Pathophysiological function of SLC25A46

In the last 2 years, a series of experiments aiming at resolving the function of SLC25A46 and the pathogenesis of *SLC25A46*-associated diseases were conducted. Primary cultures of skin fibroblasts from HMSN6B patients (including PCH or Leigh syndrome patients) have been studied to investigate the pathophysiology of the diseases. Simultaneously, mutant SLC25A46 alleles or *SLC25A46*-targeted RNA-interference molecules were transfected into common cell lines (e.g., COS-7, HeLa, HEK293T, and HCT116) to study the consequences of the mutations or protein knock-down in a homogeneous genetic background. Finally, zebrafish, murine, and bovine models have been employed to examine the pathophysiological effects of *SLC25A46* mutations *in vivo* (**Table 2**).

5.1. Function of SLC25A46 in mitochondrial dynamics

In silico analysis led to the identification of a *SLC25A46* homolog in yeast, namely *Ugo1*. The Ugo1 protein is a modified mitochondrial solute carrier expressed in the mitochondrial outer membrane that operates as a mitochondrial fusion factor and interacts physically with Mgm1 (homolog of human OPA1) and Fzo (homolog of human MFN2) [38]. A succession of studies in cells demonstrated consistently that, like Ugo1, MTCH1, and MTCH2, SLC25A46 also localizes to the mitochondrial outer membrane [17, 20, 22].

Animal species	SLC25A46 mutations	SLC25A46 proteins	Age of onset	Age of death	Optic atrophy	Peripheral neuropathy	Ataxia	Degeneration in cerebellum /brainstem	Other features	Mitochondrial dynamics
Bovine Duchesne et al. [43]	c.376C>T	p. R126C	1 mo.	Euthanasia around 2–3 mo.	–	+	+	+	Degenerative lesions both in gray matter and white matter; demyelination in certain peripheral nerves.	Elongated mitochondria with abnormal cristae.
Tg−/− FVB/N mouse Duchesne et al. [43]	Tg18: indel 12 bp; Tg26: del 75 bp	p. Val122Leu123delinsATIIYI; p.Ala108fs*159	2 w	3–4 w	–	±	+	±	Impaired growth, small intestine, thymus, spleen and liver, severe hypoglycemia; low plasma iron concentrations combined with high ferritin.	Elongated mitochondria with abnormal cristae.
atc/atc C57BL/6 J mouse Terzenidou et al. [42]	c.283C>T	p.Gln95fs*	2 w	5 w	+	+	+	+	Growth retardation, severe thymic and splenic hypoplasia, compromised Purkinje cell dendritic arborization and reduced synaptic connectivity, RGC	Atypical mitochondria in Purkinje cells.

Animal species	SLC25A46 mutations	SLC25A46 proteins	Age of onset	Age of death	Optic atrophy	Peripheral neuropathy	Ataxia	Degeneration in cerebellum /brainstem	Other features	Mitochondrial dynamics
Slc−/− B6D2 mouse Li et al. [39]	c.992_1037del	p.Leu331fs*346	2 w	2–8 w	+	+	+	+	Purkinje cell loss and dendritic abnormalities, degeneration in striatum, corpus callosum and spinal cord; axon degeneration and demyelination. aberrations, improper neuromuscular junction.	Enlarged or ring/C-shaped mitochondria.

Note: mo represents month; w the week.

Table 2. Clinical phenotypes associated with mutant SLC25A46 animal models.

Knock down of SLC25A46 in various cell lines by different research groups caused mitochondrial hyperfusion and abnormal cristae architecture visualized with fluorescent staining and electron microscopy [17, 20, 22]. In concordance, in an ultrastructural study of a SLC25A46 knock-out mouse model, we observed enlarged mitochondria with swollen cristae in Purkinje cell (PC) dendrites and sciatic nerves (**Table 2**) [39]. Hyperfused mitochondria consequent to SLC25A46 loss was unexpected because loss of Ugo1 function usually results in mitochondrial fission; however, it should be noted that strikingly similar cristae architecture abnormalities from loss of function are common to both genes [38, 40, 41]. Interestingly, in SLC25A46 mutant Purkinje cell bodies, ring-shaped or C-shaped mitochondria (a rarely reported morphology) were more commonly observed than hyperfused mitochondria [39, 42]. Furthermore, mitochondria were found to have an abnormal distribution and impaired movement within mutant Purkinje cells in a primary culture of mouse cerebellar cells [39]. These findings confirm that SLC25A46 plays an important role in the regulation of mitochondrial dynamics, including mitochondrial fusion/fission, distribution, and movement, as well as the maintenance of cristae architecture. Regarding the molecular actions of SLC25A46 in the balance of mitochondrial dynamics, recent research findings present three possible explanations: (1) SLC25A46 may act as an independent pro-fission factor; (2) SLC25A46 may serve as a regulator by interacting with mitochondrial fusion machinery, such as through an association with MFN1/2 oligomerization; and (3) SLC25A46 may regulate mitochondrial dynamics through its functions in lipid transfer between the endoplasmic reticulum (ER) and mitochondria.

In an inter-institution collaborative exploratory study employing immunoprecipitation assays and mass spectrometry analysis, there was no evidence of SLC25A46 interacting with MFN2 or OPA1 in HEK293T cells, but rather SLC25A46 was observed forming a complex with mitofilin that was independent of MFN2 [17]. Furthermore, overexpression of wild-type SLC25A46 protein led to mitochondrial fragmentation and disruption of the mitochondrial network. Thus, SLC25A46 was proposed to act as a pro-fission factor [17]. In contrast, two subsequent studies using similar immunoprecipitation approaches in patient fibroblasts and two cell lines (HEK293T with stable wild-type SLC25A46 expression and LAN5 neuronal cells) showed SLC25A46 interactions with proteins involved in fission and fusion, including MFN1/2 and OPA1, as well as with components of the MICOS (mitochondrial contact site and cristae organizing system) complex (**Figure 1**) [18, 20]. Moreover, decreased expression of SLC25A46 resulted in increased stability and oligomerization of MFN1 and MFN2 in association with mitochondria, thus promoting mitochondrial hyperfusion [18]. In SLC25A46 knock-out mice, two independent mass spectrometry studies yielded opposite results regarding the interaction between SLC25A46 and common dynamic proteins [42, 43]. Hence, although it seems reasonable that SLC25A46 would have interaction relationships with MFN1/MFN2 and the MICOS complex similar to those of Ugo1, further studies are needed to resolve its molecular mechanisms given the current conflicting results in the literature.

MFN2 tethers the ER to the mitochondrial network, suggesting that the ER may have a physical relationship with the mitochondrial network [44]. SLC25A46 has also been shown to interact with all nine components of the endoplasmic reticulum membrane complex (EMC) [18, 20], an ER protein complex recently shown to be necessary for phospholipid transfer from the ER to mitochondria in yeast. Most mitochondrial phospholipid species were altered dramatically by the loss of SLC25A46, indicating that SLC25A46 provides direct coupling of lipid flux between the ER and mitochondria at outer-inner mitochondrial membrane contacts [20]. Meanwhile, endoplasmic reticulum chaperone BiP (a.k.a. 78 kDa glucose-regulated protein), which acts at the ER-mitochondria interface under stress conditions and is considered as a major regulator of the ER, was down-regulated in *SLC25A46* knock-out mice [43]. These findings support the notion that the facilitation of lipid flux at ER contact sites may be a primary function of SLC25A46.

Studies implicating OPA1 and the MICOS complex in the maintenance of cristae architecture are compelling, but it is unclear how they may interact [45]. The observation that SLC25A46 interacts with OPA1 and MIC60, the major MICOS organizer, provides a molecular link that may integrate their functions in modulating cristae architecture [18, 20].

It now seems likely that SLC25A46 may possess multiple homeostatic functions in mitochondrial dynamics. Further studies are expected to reveal more refined details of the pathophysiological functions of SLC25A46, such as which domain interacts with dynamic proteins and which domain recognizes and communicates with the ER.

5.2. Consequences of SLC25A46 dysfunction on mitochondrial metabolism

Disorganization of cristae leads to disruption of the assembly of the respiratory supercomplexes that mediate oxidative phosphorylation, which reduces the activity of their components (i.e., respiratory complexes I–V) and, thus, diminishes respiration efficiency [46, 47]. Mitochondrial metabolism is disrupted in both patients with mutant *SLC25A46* alleles and animal models of disrupted *SLC25A46*. Fibroblasts from patients harboring mutant *SLC25A46* showed varying extents of decreased oxygen consumption rate and glycolytic shift (decreased oxygen consumption rate-to-extracellular acidification rate ratio), consistent with the increased lactate levels indicated by magnetic resonance spectroscopy (MRS) [17]. Moreover, siRNA-mediated suppression of SLC25A46 in control fibroblasts phenocopied the basal oxygen consumption defect observed in the cells of patients with mutant *SLC25A46*, confirming a specific function of SLC25A46 in respiration [20]. Given the specificity of each tissue and each cell type in responding to physiological stresses and mutations, mitochondria isolated from the cerebellum of SLC25A46 knock-out mouse displayed a remarkable decrease in the activities of respiratory complexes I–IV, and thus a dramatically reduced ATP production potential [39]. Taken together, these observations support the hypothesis of an energetic defect being a principal cause of *SLC25A46*-related neurological disease.

5.3. SLC25A46 dysfunction in pathology

Mitochondrial pathobiology has long been linked to the pathogenesis of neurodegenerative diseases, in part because neurons are highly dependent upon mitochondrial metabolism. Autopsy on a pair of deceased siblings who died due to *SLC25A46* mutations showed a very small cerebellum, as well as degenerative changes in the inferior olive nucleus. Histology of the cervical spinal cord illustrated loss and ongoing degeneration of spinal motoneurons in the medial anterior horn at all levels from the cervical to the lumbar region. Rectus femoris muscle biopsies showed severely atrophied muscle fibers of all types, without type grouping [48].

For now, most anatomical and histological analyses for *SLC25A46*-related diseases are based on animal models. Four *SLC25A46* mutant mammalian models have been discovered or designed, including a calf model and 3 mouse models with different genetic backgrounds (**Table 2**). Turning calf syndrome, a neurodegenerative disease, is characterized during massive inbreeding in cattle. Genetic study determines that this disease resulted from a single substitution in the coding region of the *SLC25A46* [43]. All affected calves manifested early onset of ataxia, especially of hind limbs, and paraparesis (2–6 weeks old). Despite symptomatic care, nervous symptoms progressed over the next months, leading to repetitive falls and ultimately resulting in permanent recumbency and inevitably euthanasia. Characteristic degenerative microscopic lesions were found in both gray matter (brainstem lateral vestibular nuclei and spinal cord thoracic nuclei) and white matter (dorsolateral and ventromedial funiculi of the spinal cord) regions of the central nervous system, as well as demyelination of some peripheral nerves [49]. Electron microscopy confirmed this neuropathy phenotype, revealing discrete demyelinating lesions and some enlarged nodes of Ranvier.

Three SLC25A46 knock-out mouse models with different genetic backgrounds, including FVB/N, C57BL/6J, and B6D2, were generated, respectively (**Table 2**). In spite of various mutation positions and sizes, three mouse lines displayed very similar phenotypes, including growth delay, progressive ataxia, optic atrophy, short life span, which recapitulated the pathological state in human. Further histopathologic studies have shown tissue- and cell-specific lesions in both the central nervous system and peripheral nervous system (**Table 2**).

Although macroscopic examination showed no overt abnormalities in the gross anatomy of mutant brain, histological staining revealed markedly reduced cerebellums, with Purkinje cells (PCs) that had stunted dendrites and were reduced in number. Degeneration (evidenced by Fluoro-Jade C dye) was selectively present in mutant PCs [39]. Examination via electron microscopy (EM) revealed that degenerated PC dendrites exhibited disorganized cytoskeleton, often containing remnants of mitochondria and other organelles. Numerous atypical mitochondria with cytoplasmic inclusions were found both in the soma and dendrites of PCs. In addition, a significant reduction in vGlut1 and vGlut2 immunoreactivity both in PCs and molecular layer indicated a paucity of glutamatergic synapses in mutant mice [42]. Apart from PCs, degenerative signals were also aggregated in the vestibular nucleus of brainstem, deep cerebellar nuclei, the striatum, the corpus callosum, and the spinal cord, but not in other parts of the brain [39]. The neurodegeneration was associated with astrogliosis and microgliosis in the cerebellum and spinal cord, indicating high levels of neuroinflammation [39, 42]. These observations suggest that although *SLC25A46* mRNA is transcribed in most neural tissues, SLC25A46 may have a tissue- or cell-specific function. Interestingly, mice with conditional knock-out *MFN2* or *DRP1* mutations showed a similar phenomenon, with major changes in cerebellar Purkinje cells, whereas granule cells seemed to be spared [50]. It is not yet known why specific neurons are selectively affected by mitochondrial dysfunction. It could be that a large neuronal size makes particular neurons susceptible; Purkinje cells are one of the largest neuron types in the brain with long axons and extremely extensive dendritic branches. Their complex architecture requires the transport and distribution of highly organized organelles, including mitochondria.

Aged SLC25A46 mutant mice displayed enhanced hind limb clasping reflex and muscle atrophy, suggesting potential peripheral neuropathy. Acquiring compound muscle action potentials (CMAPs) reduced in mutant sciatic nerve measured by electromyography (EMG) *in vivo* [39]. Mutant peripheral nerves exhibited sporadic degenerative lesions with local macrophages containing lipid debris and signs of demyelination. In addition, the size of individual endplates in mutant mice was significantly reduced. Retarded neuromuscular junction maturation and improper innervation, early hallmarks of CMT2D, were also documented in mutant muscle [42]. All of these alterations are indicative of peripheral neuropathy.

Optical coherence tomography (OCT) scanning on retina for live mice revealed that although the optic discs were grossly normal in terms of retinal appearance, retinas were thinner in aged SLC25A46 mutant mice [39]. Further quantitative measurements indicated that ganglion cell complex (GCC) thicknesses, which includes the nerve fiber layer (NFL), ganglion cell layer (GCL), and inner plexiform layer (IPL), were significantly reduced in adult mutant mice. Retinal and these reductions were associated with retinal ganglion cell loss and atypically small optic nerve axons with reduced neurofilament expression, as well as some axons that exhibited signs of degeneration and demyelination [39, 42]. Pax6+ and GAD65+ GABAergic amacrine cells—both of which form synapses with retinal ganglion cells—were also significantly reduced. These pathological changes are in line with the phenotypic features of ADOA.

Ultrastructural studies revealed dysmorphic mitochondria in both the central and peripheral nervous systems. Numerous enlarged and round mitochondria with abnormal cristae were found in Purkinje cell dendrites, while ring- or C-shaped mitochondria were commonly observed in soma. Peripheral nerve axons also had abnormal round, fused, and aggregated mitochondria in myelinated and non-myelinated fibers [39, 43].

Given the degeneration in long peripheral axons and distal optic nerves of SLC25A46 knock-out animal models, the aforementioned findings support the idea that neurons with long axons or complicated dendrites are more sensitive to abnormal mitochondrial dynamics. Similar to the findings in mutant Purkinje cells, this sensitivity could also be due to the impaired transport of hyperfused mitochondria along axons and dendrites, probably due to their abnormal size and/or reduced ATP availability in the distal portions of long axons secondary to mitochondrial dysfunction. Further studies are needed to clarify this point.

6. Conclusion

SLC25A46 plays a critical role in mitochondrial dynamics and the maintenance of mitochondrial cristae, which are particularly important in neurodevelopment and neurodegeneration. Loss of SLC25A46 function causes a wide spectrum of neurodegenerative diseases, including optic atrophy, peripheral neuropathy, progressive ataxia, Leigh syndrome, and lethal congenital pontocerebellar hypoplasia. In SLC25A46-related neurodegenerative diseases, phenotype severity correlates strongly with the magnitude of SLC25A46 level deficit observed.

Acknowledgements

This work was supported by the Center for Pediatric Genomics at the Cincinnati Children's Hospital, a grant from the National Institutes of Health (1R01EY026609-01) to Taosheng Huang, and a grant from the National Natural Science Foundation of China (81470299) to Zhuo Li.

Conflict of interest

The authors declare that they have no conflicts of interest.

Author details

Zhuo Li[1,2], Jesse Slone[1], Lingqian Wu[2] and Taosheng Huang[1,3]*

*Address all correspondence to: taosheng.huang@cchmc.org

1 Division of Human Genetics, Cincinnati Children's Hospital Medical Center, Cincinnati, OH, USA

2 Center for Medical Genetics, School of Life Sciences, Central South University, Changsha, Hunan, China

3 Human Aging Research Institute, Nanchang University, Nanchang, Jiangxi, China

References

[1] Kann O, Kovacs R. Mitochondria and neuronal activity. American Journal of Physiology-Cell Physiology. 2007;**292**(2):C641-C657

[2] Chen H, Chan DC. Mitochondrial dynamics–fusion, fission, movement, and mitophagy–in neurodegenerative diseases. Human Molecular Genetics. 2009;**18**(R2):R169-R176

[3] Twig G, Hyde B, Shirihai OS. Mitochondrial fusion, fission and autophagy as a quality control axis: The bioenergetic view. Biochimica et Biophysica Acta. 2008;**1777**(9):1092-1097

[4] Su B, Wang X, Bonda D, Perry G, Smith M, Zhu X. Abnormal mitochondrial dynamics—A novel therapeutic target for Alzheimer's disease? Molecular Neurobiology. 2010;41(2-3): 87-96

[5] Zuchner S, Mersiyanova IV, Muglia M, Bissar-Tadmouri N, Rochelle J, Dadali EL, et al. Mutations in the mitochondrial GTPase mitofusin 2 cause Charcot-Marie-tooth neuropathy type 2A. Nature Genetics. 2004;36(5):449-451

[6] Lawson VH, Graham BV, Flanigan KM. Clinical and electrophysiologic features of CMT2A with mutations in the mitofusin 2 gene. Neurology. 2005;65(2):197-204

[7] Cartoni R, Martinou JC. Role of mitofusin 2 mutations in the physiopathology of Charcot-Marie-tooth disease type 2A. Experimental Neurology. 2009;218(2):268-273

[8] Olichon A, Guillou E, Delettre C, Landes T, Arnaune-Pelloquin L, Emorine LJ, et al. Mitochondrial dynamics and disease, OPA1. Biochimica et Biophysica Acta. 2006;1763(5-6): 500-509

[9] Alexander C, Votruba M, Pesch UE, Thiselton DL, Mayer S, Moore A, et al. OPA1, encoding a dynamin-related GTPase, is mutated in autosomal dominant optic atrophy linked to chromosome 3q28. Nature Genetics. 2000;26(2):211-215

[10] Delettre C, Lenaers G, Griffoin JM, Gigarel N, Lorenzo C, Belenguer P, et al. Nuclear gene OPA1, encoding a mitochondrial dynamin-related protein, is mutated in dominant optic atrophy. Nature Genetics. 2000;26(2):207-210

[11] Waterham HR, Koster J, van Roermund CW, Mooyer PA, Wanders RJ, Leonard JV. A lethal defect of mitochondrial and peroxisomal fission. New England Journal of Medicine. 2007;356(17):1736-1741

[12] Cassereau J, Codron P, Funalot B. Inherited peripheral neuropathies due to mitochondrial disorders. Revue Neurologique. 2014;170(5):366-374

[13] Sajic M. Mitochondrial dynamics in peripheral neuropathies. Antioxidants & Redox Signaling. 2014;21(4):601-620

[14] Schwarz TL. Mitochondrial trafficking in neurons. Cold Spring Harbor perspectives in biology. 2013;5(6):a011304

[15] Turnbull HE, Lax NZ, Diodato D, Ansorge O, Turnbull DM. The mitochondrial brain: From mitochondrial genome to neurodegeneration. Biochimica et Biophysica Acta. 2010; 1802(1):111-121

[16] Archer SL. Mitochondrial dynamics—Mitochondrial fission and fusion in human diseases. New England Journal of Medicine. 2013;369(23):2236-2251

[17] Abrams AJ, Hufnagel RB, Rebelo A, Zanna C, Patel N, Gonzalez MA, et al. Mutations in SLC25A46, encoding a UGO1-like protein, cause an optic atrophy spectrum disorder. Nature Genetics. 2015;47(8):926-932

[18] Steffen J, Vashisht AA, Wan J, Jen JC, Claypool SM, Wohlschlegel JA, et al. Rapid degradation of mutant SLC25A46 by the ubiquitin-proteasome system results in MFN1/2-mediated hyperfusion of mitochondria. Molecular Biology of the Cell. 2017; **28**(5):600-612

[19] Charlesworth G, Balint B, Mencacci NE, Carr L, Wood NW, Bhatia KP. SLC25A46 mutations underlie progressive myoclonic ataxia with optic atrophy and neuropathy. Movement Disorders. 2016;**31**(8):1249-1251

[20] Janer A, Prudent J, Paupe V, Fahiminiya S, Majewski J, Sgarioto N, et al. SLC25A46 is required for mitochondrial lipid homeostasis and cristae maintenance and is responsible for Leigh syndrome. EMBO Molecular Medicine. 2016;**8**(9):1019-1038

[21] Nguyen M, Boesten I, Hellebrekers D, Mulder-den Hartog NM, de Coo I, Smeets H, et al. Novel pathogenic SLC25A46 splice-site mutation causes an optic atrophy spectrum disorder. Clinical Genetics. 2017;**91**(1):121-125

[22] Wan J, Steffen J, Yourshaw M, Mamsa H, Andersen E, Rudnik-Schoneborn S, et al. Loss of function of SLC25A46 causes lethal congenital pontocerebellar hypoplasia. Brain: A Journal of Neurology. 2016;**139**(11):2877-2890

[23] Hammer MB, Ding J, Mochel F, Eleuch-Fayache G, Charles P, Coutelier M, et al. SLC25A46 mutations associated with autosomal recessive cerebellar ataxia in north African families. Neuro-Degenerative Diseases. 2017;**17**(4-5):208-212

[24] Braunisch MC, Gallwitz H, Abicht A, Diebold I, Holinski-Feder E, Van Maldergem L, et al. Extension of the phenotype of biallelic loss-of-function mutations in SLC25A46 to the severe form of pontocerebellar hypoplasia type I. Clinical Genetics. 2018;**93**(2):255-265

[25] van Dijk T, Rudnik-Schoneborn S, Senderek J, Hajmousa G, Mei H, Dusl M, et al. Pontocerebellar hypoplasia with spinal muscular atrophy (PCH1): Identification of SLC25A46 mutations in the original Dutch PCH1 family. Brain. 2017;**140**(8):e46

[26] Sulaiman RA, Patel N, Alsharif H, Arold ST, Alkuraya FS. A novel mutation in SLC25A46 causes optic atrophy and progressive limb spasticity, with no cerebellar atrophy or axonal neuropathy. Clinical Genetics. 2017;**92**(2):230-231

[27] Haitina T, Lindblom J, Renstrom T, Fredriksson R. Fourteen novel human members of mitochondrial solute carrier family 25 (SLC25) widely expressed in the central nervous system. Genomics. 2006;**88**(6):779-790

[28] Palmieri F. The mitochondrial transporter family SLC25: Identification, properties and physiopathology. Molecular Aspects of Medicine. 2013;**34**(2-3):465-484

[29] Monne M, Palmieri F, Kunji ER. The substrate specificity of mitochondrial carriers: Mutagenesis revisited. Molecular Membrane Biology. 2013;**30**(2):149-159

[30] Palmieri F. Mitochondrial transporters of the SLC25 family and associated diseases: A review. Journal of Inherited Metabolic Disease. 2014;**37**(4):565-575

[31] Robinson AJ, Kunji ER. Mitochondrial carriers in the cytoplasmic state have a common substrate binding site. Proceedings of the National Academy of Sciences of the United States of America. 2006;**103**(8):2617-2622

[32] Kunji ER, Robinson AJ. The conserved substrate binding site of mitochondrial carriers. Biochimica et Biophysica Acta. 2006;**1757**(9-10):1237-1248

[33] Palmieri F, Monne M. Discoveries, metabolic roles and diseases of mitochondrial carriers: A review. Biochimica et Biophysica Acta. 2016;**1863**(10):2362-2378

[34] Yu-Wai-Man P, Griffiths PG, Hudson G, Chinnery PF. Inherited mitochondrial optic neuropathies. Journal of Medical Genetics. 2009;**46**(3):145-158

[35] Zuchner S, Vance JM. Emerging pathways for hereditary axonopathies. Journal of Molecular Medicine. 2005;**83**(12):935-943

[36] Feely SM, Laura M, Siskind CE, Sottile S, Davis M, Gibbons VS, et al. MFN2 mutations cause severe phenotypes in most patients with CMT2A. Neurology. 2011;**76**(20):1690-1696

[37] Fahrner JA, Liu R, Perry MS, Klein J, Chan DC. A novel de novo dominant negative mutation in DNM1L impairs mitochondrial fission and presents as childhood epileptic encephalopathy. American Journal of Medical Genetics Part A. 2016;**170**(8):2002-2011

[38] Sesaki H, Jensen RE. Ugo1p links the Fzo1p and Mgm1p GTPases for mitochondrial fusion. Journal of Biological Chemistry. 2004;**279**(27):28298-28303

[39] Li Z, Peng Y, Hufnagel RB, Hu YC, Zhao C, Queme LF, et al. Loss of SLC25A46 causes neurodegeneration by affecting mitochondrial dynamics and energy production in mice. Human Molecular Genetics. 2017;**26**(19):3776-3791

[40] Sesaki H, Jensen RE. UGO1 encodes an outer membrane protein required for mitochondrial fusion. Journal of Cell Biology. 2001;**152**(6):1123-1134

[41] Hoppins S, Horner J, Song C, McCaffery JM, Nunnari J. Mitochondrial outer and inner membrane fusion requires a modified carrier protein. Journal of Cell Biology. 2009;**184**(4):569-581

[42] Terzenidou ME, Segklia A, Kano T, Papastefanaki F, Karakostas A, Charalambous M, et al. Novel insights into SLC25A46-related pathologies in a genetic mouse model. PLoS Genetics. 2017;**13**(4):e1006656

[43] Duchesne A, Vaiman A, Castille J, Beauvallet C, Gaignard P, Floriot S, et al. Bovine and murine models highlight novel roles for SLC25A46 in mitochondrial dynamics and metabolism, with implications for human and animal health. PLoS Genetics. 2017;**13**(4):e1006597

[44] Leal NS, Schreiner B, Pinho CM, Filadi R, Wiehager B, Karlstrom H, et al. Mitofusin-2 knockdown increases ER-mitochondria contact and decreases amyloid beta-peptide production. Journal of Cellular and Molecular Medicine. 2016;**20**(9):1686-1695

[45] van, der Laan M, Horvath SE, Pfanner N. Mitochondrial contact site and cristae organizing system. Current Opinion in Cell Biology. 2016;**41**:33-42

[46] Friedman JR, Mourier A, Yamada J, McCaffery JM, Nunnari J. MICOS coordinates with respiratory complexes and lipids to establish mitochondrial inner membrane architecture. eLife. 2015;**4**:e07739

[47] Cogliati S, Frezza C, Soriano ME, Varanita T, Quintana-Cabrera R, Corrado M, et al. Mitochondrial cristae shape determines respiratory chain supercomplexes assembly and respiratory efficiency. Cell. 2013;**155**(1):160-171

[48] Barth PG. Pontocerebellar hypoplasias. An overview of a group of inherited neurodegenerative disorders with fetal onset. Brain and Development. 1993;**15**(6):411-422

[49] Timsit E, Albaric O, Colle MA, Costiou P, Cesbron N, Bareille N, et al. Clinical and histopathologic characterization of a central and peripheral axonopathy in rouge-des-pres (Maine Anjou) calves. Journal of Veterinary Internal Medicine. 2011;**25**(2):386-392

[50] Chen H, McCaffery JM, Chan DC. Mitochondrial fusion protects against neurodegeneration in the cerebellum. Cell. 2007;**130**(3):548-562